Your
BODY,
Your
HEALTH
CARE

Your
BODY,
Your
HEALTH
CARE

JEFFREY A. SINGER, MD

Print ISBN: 978-1-964524-45-0
eBook ISBN: 978-1-964524-46-7

Cover: Faceout Studio.

Imagery licensed from Shutterstock.

Library of Congress Cataloging Number: 2024059083

Printed in the United States of America.

CATO INSTITUTE
1000 Massachusetts Ave. NW
Washington, DC 20001
www.cato.org

To autonomous adults everywhere.

CONTENTS

PART ONE
FIRST PRINCIPLES

PART TWO
AUTONOMY MEANS THE RIGHT TO CHOOSE YOUR
HEALTH CARE PROVIDER

PART THREE
AUTONOMY MEANS ENDING
THE GOVERNMENT'S POWER OVER
WHAT MEDICATIONS PEOPLE CAN CONSUME

PART FOUR
AUTONOMY MEANS THE RIGHT
TO SELF-MEDICATE FOR *ANY* REASON

PART FIVE
AUTONOMY MEANS THE RIGHT
TO SEEK HARM REDUCTION

PART SIX
DEFENDING AUTONOMY

As a general surgeon, when patients consult me for health problems and I determine that an operation would help solve their problem, I explain, in plain English and avoiding medical jargon, what the operation entails. I tell them why the operation is necessary to solve their problem. I tell them the risks and benefits of the procedure and make them aware of the pros and cons of surgical and nonsurgical alternatives to the proposed operation. I don't proceed to operate without their informed consent. While I do all this out of respect for my patients' autonomy, my profession's ethics also require me to do this. Nowadays, civil tort case law requires it as well.

The doctrine of "informed consent"—that individuals have a right to refuse whatever medical or surgical treatment they choose, even if doing so will harm them—is a relatively modern development. A little over 100 years ago, society commonly accepted that doctors could do whatever they perceived was in the best interests of their patients, regardless of a patient's wishes or priorities.

Things began to change in 1908 when Mary Schloendorff, a patient at New York Hospital, consented to a diagnostic examination under anesthesia for a suspected uterine tumor. She explicitly stated that she did not want to undergo an operation while under anesthesia but instead wanted to discuss the findings with the doctor and later decide about surgery. Despite her instructions, the examining surgeon diagnosed a uterine fibroid tumor and proceeded to remove it. Schloendorff subsequently sustained postoperative complications that ultimately caused gangrene in her left arm, which required surgeons to amputate several of her fingers.[1]

Schloendorff sued the Society of New York Hospital for assault and won on the merits. After the defendants appealed the decision, New York Appeals Court Judge Benjamin Cardozo (later a US Supreme Court Justice), in 1914, wrote for the majority:

> In the case at hand, the wrong complained of is not merely negligence. It is trespass. *Every human being of adult years and sound mind has a right to determine what shall be done with his own body; and a surgeon who performs an operation without his patient's consent, commits an assault, for which he is liable in damages.* This is true except in cases of emergency where the patient is unconscious and where it is necessary to operate before consent can be obtained.... [Schloendorff] had never consented to become a patient for any purpose other than an examination under ether.... she had forbidden the operation.[2]

It took decades for informed consent to become a hallmark of medical ethics. Even into the 1970s, many doctors admitted to withholding terminal cancer diagnoses from their patients.[3] Nowadays, the patient-doctor relationship has largely shifted from one of medical paternalism and patient acquiescence to what bioethicist Daniel Sokol calls a "leveled partnership" in which the medical profession respects patient autonomy and the government punishes providers who violate the doctrine of informed consent.[4]

While informed consent and respect for autonomy govern how health care practitioners interact with their patients, this new ethos is absent when it comes to the government asserting authority over adults' health decisions. The government dictates what kinds of health professionals adults may consult. It determines what medicines adults may purchase and under which circumstances they may consume them. It bans adults from ingesting substances or engaging in activities that the government decides are unhealthful, regardless of individual risk-benefit priorities. It does all this because the government assumes it knows what is in adults' best interest. In summary, every day the government treats all adults the way that Mary Schloendorff's doctors treated her.

In the following pages, I want to inform you about how lawmakers and policymakers at all levels of government have failed to heed Judge Cardozo's pronouncement that "every human being of adult years and sound mind has a right to determine what shall be done with his own body." I hope to expose the harmful unintended consequences of this paternalism. Finally, I want to point out roads leading to a future where the government respects the autonomy and rights of all adults.

PART ONE

First Principles

CHAPTER 1

Autonomy, Informed Consent, and the Right to Self-Medicate

A central tenet of the liberal tradition is that every individual has autonomy, or what philosopher John Christman calls "the capacity to be one's own person, to live one's life according to reasons and motives that are taken as one's own and not the product of manipulative or distorting external forces, to be in this way independent."[1]

In the context of the clinician-patient relationship, autonomy means that health care practitioners must respect their patients' decisionmaking capacity and their right to make their own decisions regarding their care, regardless of practitioners' recommendations. Autonomy means a patient has both liberty and agency (the capacity to act purposefully).

We take respect for patient autonomy and the doctrine of informed consent for granted in modern times. Yet countless people died or suffered great harm over the centuries before these precepts became the norm. And, while autonomy is now an inalienable feature of the relationship between people and their health care providers, it receives short shrift in the relationship between people and their government. The context might be different, but the principle is the same.

In *Principles of Biomedical Ethics*, Tom L. Beauchamp and James F. Childress contend that a patient's autonomy is paramount. They stress that health care providers must not coerce or manipulate patients into making health care choices that go against their interests or desires.[2] Requiring clinicians to obtain informed consent from their patients before performing any tests or procedures is an indispensable component of respect for patients' autonomy.

As mentioned in the introduction, the landmark New York Appeals Court case *Schloendorff v. Society of New York Hospital* established patient autonomy as a legal principle. But *Schloendorff* was the culmination of other cases that involved doctors performing procedures on patients without their consent. Most notable among these are *Mohr v. Williams* and *Pratt v. Davis*, both in 1905.[3] In *Mohr*, a surgeon, Cornelius Williams, changed his mind when Anna Mohr was under anesthesia and decided to operate on her left ear instead of the right one. She had consented only to surgery on the right ear. Williams's decision left Mohr with impaired hearing in both ears. In the latter case, Edwin H. Pratt, a surgeon, performed a hysterectomy on Parmelia Davis to treat her epilepsy, which many doctors once believed was uterine in origin, without her consent.[4] The courts decided both cases in favor of the plaintiffs.[5]

In *Mohr v. Williams*, the Minnesota Supreme Court concluded that an operation that is performed without the consent of the patient is wrongful, except in a life-threatening situation, which was not the case with Anna Mohr.[6] In *Pratt v. Davis*, the court elaborated further:

> Under a free government at least, the citizen's first and greatest right, which underlies all others—the fight to the inviolability of his person, in other words, his right to himself. . .[7]

The opinions rendered in these earlier cases presaged Benjamin Cardozo's more explicit and timeless 1914 paean to autonomy in *Schloendorff*:

> Every human being of adult years and sound mind has a right to determine what shall be done with his own body. . .[8]

The horrors made public by the Nuremberg war crimes trials following the end of World War II further fueled support for the doctrine of informed consent. *Canterbury v. Spence* (1972) elaborated on informed consent in the case law by establishing that clinicians must explain not only what a procedure is and why they believe it is necessary, but also the procedure's risks—including complications—and its benefits. The DC Circuit Court of Appeals concluded that doctors engage in manipulation if they deprive patients of this information, thus indirectly coercing them.[9]

Just as health care providers violate their patients' autonomy by manipulating or coercing them, the government violates autonomy when it deprives them of their choice of health care provider, denies them access to a drug or therapy, or forbids and even punishes them for consuming products or engaging in activities of which the government disapproves.

Nonadults, the Mentally Impaired, and Autonomy

Children, minors, and the mentally impaired lack the mental and cognitive skills required to exercise full autonomy. Philosophers and legal scholars have debated this complex and thorny issue for centuries. From the natural-rights perspective, many philosophers tie human rights to rationality and the ability to live and make decisions independently that it bestows.[10]

Parents are responsible for bringing their children into existence. Until a child's faculties develop from a state of nonrational dependence to a state of rational independence, parents have a moral obligation to attend to their children's welfare and to prepare them for autonomous adulthood. As legal scholar Eugene Volokh writes:

> Children, up to a certain age, need someone to make decisions
> for them, with an eye towards putting them in the best position to

exercise their liberty once the children grow up. Someone needs
both to shield them from dangers that may keep them from surviving
to adulthood (disease, accidental death, starvation, criminal attack),
and to positively provide them the things they need (education,
self-control, and the like).

That someone can be the parents, or some interested third party—in
principle, perhaps a family member or someone else, but (system-
ically) likely government officials. But parents, generally speaking,
are much more likely to love the child and to know the child than
any third party would.[11]

The government recognizes and supports the authority of parents
to exercise fiduciary authority over their children until they reach an
age when they can exercise rational independence. However, parental
authority is not boundless, and the state may step into that role if parents neglect, harm, or otherwise exercise their authority in bad faith.
For instance, parents may not abuse their children, sell them to other
people, or refuse to let them have lifesaving procedures. Similar principles apply to people who have cognitive or mental disabilities that
don't let them achieve rational independence.

The tension between parents' authority and their moral obligations
to their children is at the center of many contentious issues that legal
and ethical scholars have long debated. Health care practitioners
sometimes are caught in the crossfire when faced with therapeutic
dilemmas. Examples include parents barring their children from medical treatment due to their religious beliefs, performing "normalizing
surgery" on infants born with "intersex disorders," and permitting
irreversible "gender-affirming" treatments and procedures on young
children and adolescents.[12]

These issues are too complex to address in this book adequately.
The book's remaining pages will refer only to the autonomy of

rational adults. In that regard, as I will discuss in later chapters, it is unwise for policymakers to target policies at adults based on concerns about children. Many laws prohibit children from indulging in various adult activities or substances for good reason. Policymakers should resist the temptation to ban adults from them in order to prevent children from gaining access. Such bans assault adults' autonomy.

The Right to Self-Medicate

The notion that competent adults have the right to self-medicate is a corollary of the doctrine of informed consent. The doctrine asserts that individuals have a right to refuse whatever medical treatment they choose, even if doing so will harm them. The right to self-medicate is the idea that individuals likewise have a right to ingest whatever medicines and use whatever medical treatments they choose, even if doing so will harm them.

To British philosopher John Stuart Mill, only the affected individual is best qualified to judge whether a risk is worth taking because no other person cares more about that individual's best interest. Even if patients make the wrong decisions, Mill maintained that society should regard them as if they are the experts about what is in their best interests because they have insights into their own priorities for well-being and happiness that no other person can have. Mill argued against the government blocking people from purchasing certain drugs unless they obtained a physician's prescription, arguing that it interferes with patients' choices and may make certain drugs more expensive or more difficult for them to get.[13]

The right to self-medicate is integral to self-ownership and autonomy. Philosophy professor Jessica Flanigan, who specializes in bioethics, writes that respect for the right to self-medicate is so embedded in the liberal tradition that 18th-century political thinkers would regularly affirm it:

> For example, Thomas Jefferson assumes that self-medication is a fundamental right in arguing for freedom of conscience when he wrote, "Reason and free enquiry are the only effectual agents against error. Give a loose to them; they will support the true religion, by bringing every false one to their tribunal. . . . If it be restrained now, the present corruptions will be protected, and new ones encouraged. Was the government to prescribe to us our medicine and diet, our bodies would be in such keeping as our souls are now."[14]

Flanigan argues that government-mandated premarket approval and prescription requirements are forms of coercive medical paternalism that interfere with individual autonomy as much as when doctors lie to patients about the patients' diagnoses, prognoses, or treatment options or perform unauthorized procedures on them:

> Paternalism is just as wrong at the pharmacy as it is in the doctor's office. Medical autonomy is an important value in both contexts, so states should protect patients' rights against unwanted medical interventions from physicians and from unwanted limits on access by public officials. Both informed consent requirements and rights of self-medication will permit people to make decisions that their physicians would advise against.[15]

Flanigan identifies two areas where the government may ethically restrict the ability to self-medicate. One is antibiotics. Consumers who use antibiotics indiscriminately promote the development of antibiotic-resistant organisms, which can potentially expose others to the risk of harm or even death from infectious diseases.[16] This is what economists call a *negative externality*.[17]

The other area pertains to children and to adults with severe cognitive disabilities who have a capacity for autonomy not dissimilar to that of children. Such individuals are unable to make medical decisions in accordance with the doctrine of informed consent and therefore cannot claim the right to self-medication. Flanigan argues that it is therefore ethically permissible to restrict their access to medications.[18]

The doctrine of informed consent and the right to self-medicate are inextricably linked. Any argument that individuals do not have a right to self-medicate necessarily undermines the doctrine of informed consent. It is impossible to infringe on one without threatening the other. If one is valid, so is the other. If one supports the doctrine of informed consent, one must logically respect the right to self-medicate. Both informed consent and the right to self-medicate are features of autonomy.

CHAPTER 2

Licensing and Scope of Practice Laws

To illustrate a point, consider the following scenario. Arizona, the state where I reside, granted me a medical license more than 40 years ago. A few years later, I became board-certified in general surgery and have been practicing in that specialty ever since. After 40-plus years of practicing surgery, suppose I need a new challenge. I have been reading and taking weekend courses in psychiatry and have developed a keen interest in the field. So, I decide to switch specialties and change the sign on my office door from "general surgery" to "psychiatry" and spread the word in the community that there is a new psychiatrist in the area. The government allows me to do this. Offering patients psychiatric help is well within a physician's scope of practice. All the medical specialties and subspecialties fall within that scope.

Next, I determine that it would help to grow my psychiatry practice if I sought psychiatric consulting privileges at the nearby private, non-profit hospital where I perform operations. In most hospitals, physicians seeking new practice privileges or wishing to expand existing ones must go before a medical staff credentials committee. The hospital committee asks me where I did my psychiatry residency and whether I was board-certified. When I tell the committee that I have not completed a psychiatry residency and am not board-certified, they reject my application. Most hospitals these days require medical staff applicants to complete a specialty residency at a minimum, and many require those applicants to have a specialty board certification in order to join the hospital staff.

Then, I contact the various health plans that list me as a surgical specialist on their provider panels and ask them to change my listing to that of mental health provider. The health plans' credentialing staff ask me where I did my psychiatry residency and if I was board-certified. When I give them the answer, the credentialing officers reply that their plans only include residency-trained specialists, preferably board-certified, on their provider panels.

Undeterred, I next contact my malpractice insurance provider to request that they update my coverage to include psychiatric malpractice. I get the same questions from the insurance company that I got from the hospital and health plan credentialing people. When I give them the same answer I gave the others, the insurance company denies my request for the same reasons that the hospital and health plans did, but offers to continue covering me for surgical malpractice if I abandon the idea of switching my specialty to psychiatry.

Under state law, I can still practice psychiatry in my office. However, the nearby hospital won't let me consult there, private health plans won't include me on their mental health provider list, and liability insurance companies won't cover me for psychiatric malpractice. The hospital, the health plans, and the liability insurance company are all part of the private sector. It is in their best interests to screen me to protect their risks and reputations. The fact that I have a state license only tells the public that I graduated from an accredited medical school, passed the standardized test, completed at least one year of residency, and do not have a felony conviction on my record. But the other organizations do the same screening.

As the above scenario illustrates, a state physician's license is a less rigorous quality signal than what private certification organizations provide. However, it protects incumbent physicians from competition from new entrants to the field.

Earning a Living: Government Permission Required

The Tenth Amendment to the US Constitution reserves to the states police powers to make laws for the public health and welfare. Most lawmakers in this country enact laws at the state and local level under that authority.[1] For over a century, state governments—assuming they know best—have been deciding what kinds of health professionals to allow patients to seek advice and care from. Every state has laws that block patients from accessing health care providers that the government has not licensed. State governments also determine health professionals' scope of practice. States limit the range of services that patients may seek from various health professionals, even when professionals have the expertise to offer those services.

This wasn't always the case. Physicians were the first health care professionals that state governments restricted patients from seeing. Today, all 50 states and the District of Columbia require physicians to graduate from an accredited medical school, pass a three-step standardized national exam, and complete at least one year of postgraduate training, called "residency," to get a license.[2] States do not require licensed physicians to become certified by a specialty board—for example, the American Board of Surgery—to receive a license to practice.[3] Of all the health professions, state governments grant physicians the broadest scope of practice.

In the early days of our republic, the medical profession envied the respect and social status enjoyed by their European counterparts. Many local medical societies lobbied their state legislatures to license the profession, hoping it would enhance its reputation and exclusivity. Several state legislatures obliged. However, in most cases states did not enforce the licensing laws, and a state license served as no more than a seal of approval. With the advent of the Jacksonian era, many lawmakers considered licensure ideologically offensive, even when unenforced. They disdained efforts by medical professionals to establish exclusive privileges and create licensed monopolies. Many so-called irregular physicians lobbied for their repeal. There was a dramatic decline in the number of states that required professional licensing between 1830 and 1860.[4]

By the 1870s, several schools of medical thought were competing for patients, with no restrictions on entry into the field. Medical professionals established the American Medical Association (AMA) in 1847 to improve medical education, lengthen the study period before graduation, and promote state licensing.[5] The AMA established a Committee on Medical Education, renamed the Council on Medical Education in 1904, which accredited medical schools. In 1919, the Council on Medical Education joined with another organization, the Association of American Medical Colleges (AAMC), which was founded in 1876, to conduct joint medical school inspections. Then in 1942, the two organizations created the Liaison Committee on Medical Education, which government licensing boards use to this day to determine if an applicant for a license graduated from an accredited medical school.[6]

It took several decades for the AMA to achieve its goal. By coordinating a network of state chapters that lobbied their legislatures, every state and the District of Columbia eventually licensed physicians. Initially, members of each state's chapter of the AMA dominated their respective state licensing boards. With time, board membership grew more diverse, but to this day, state medical associations still heavily influence the licensing boards. And the licensing requirements are practically uniform among the states.

The medical profession promoted licensing to create exclusivity and to enhance the reputation and income of its members.

Recruiting the government to confer monopoly status does not necessarily encourage sex or racial discrimination. However, licensing schemes can have pernicious effects or be used for nefarious purposes. For example, the AMA House of Delegates voted in 1868 to allow women physicians to become members and left it up to state chapters to decide whether to admit black physicians, stipulating that "local medical societies should have a right to enact segregationist or sexist admission standards without interference from the national society."[7] The AMA refused to recognize the National Medical Association, an integrated medical society that was composed of physicians from Howard University and the Freedman's Hospital in the District of Columbia.

Writing in the *AMA Journal of Ethics*, bioethicist Robert B. Baker states:

> The AMA's policy of tolerating racial exclusion was pivotal in creating a two-tier system of medicine in the American South and border states—racially divided, separate, and unequal. Within a decade African American medical societies were founded as an alternative. In 1895 these societies banded together to form an African American alternative to the AMA, the National Medical Association (NMA).[8]

This remained the policy of the AMA until the 1960s.

In 1910, educator Abraham Flexner issued a report, *Medical Education in the United States and Canada*, commissioned by the AMA and the Carnegie Foundation. The report, which came to be known as the Flexner Report, sought to standardize and improve medical education in the United States and Canada. The AMA Council on Medical Education endorsed and adopted its recommendations and transformed medical education into what exists today.

This forced the closure of many medical schools and reduced the physician supply. In 1910, there were 131 accredited medical schools in the United States. By 1923, that number had dropped by about half, to 66. Five of the seven black medical schools that existed before the adoption of the Flexner Report's recommendations closed by 1923. Only Howard University School of Medicine in Washington, DC, and Meharry Medical College in Nashville, Tennessee, remained.

Paul Starr writes:

> Blacks also faced outright exclusion from internships and from hospital privileges at all but a few institutions. The scarcity of opportunities for training and practice had material impact. In 1930 only one of every 3,000 black Americans was a doctor, and in the Deep South, the situation was even worse—in Mississippi, blacks had one doctor for every 14,634 persons.[9]

Medical licensing laws also reduced opportunities for women. Starr explains:

> As places in medical school became more scarce, schools that previously had liberal policies toward women increasingly excluded them. Administrators justified outright discrimination against qualified women candidates on the grounds that they would not continue to practice after marriage. For the next half of the century after 1910, except for wartime, the schools maintained quotas limiting women to about 5 percent of medical school admissions.[10]

Licensing laws also impede the free flow of health care providers across state lines, a feature that became an acute problem during the coronavirus pandemic of 2020–2021. Governments blocked patients in dire need of health care services from seeking care from other states' licensed providers who were willing to travel to their state. Many states suspended state license requirements during the public health emergency, allowing patients to seek care from health professionals holding licenses in other states.[11]

Over the decades, other health professions have followed the medical profession's example and sought state licensure. Advances in scientific knowledge and technology allowed for the organic development of new health professions, including many with narrower or different portfolios of medical expertise than physicians. Many members organized educational and credentialing organizations as these professions matured in order to enhance professional knowledge and standards. Several members of these new professions—for example, podiatrists, optometrists, and physical therapists—then lobbied their respective state lawmakers, seeking licensure.

The various health professions regularly battle before state lawmakers over concerns about their scope of practice. Some entrenched incumbents jealously guard the scope of practice their licenses permit, resisting efforts by other professions to encroach on their domain. Each tries to persuade lawmakers to narrow the range of services patients may seek from competing professions. In some cases, representatives of unlicensed health professions with scopes of practice that overlap the licensed professions request state licensing to avoid being prosecuted under the other professions' licensing provisions. For example, naturopaths, chiropractors, optometrists, and podiatrists sought licensing to avoid prosecution for practicing medicine without a license.[12] In this way, professional licensing begets more professional licensing. None of the professions consider patient autonomy. Patients didn't ask lawmakers to license health professionals. Patients have little to no say in the matter.

When other people make decisions about health and happiness for us, the choices are no longer ours. When licensing and scope of practice laws dictate the number and types of health professions patients may legally access, shortages and surpluses may develop. This can impact the distribution of health care resources and potentially hinder innovation in the field.

A report from the Association of American Medical Colleges projects a shortage of up to 86,000 physicians, including approximately 40,000 primary care physicians, by 2036.[13] A 2020 study published in *Human Resources for Health* projects that the three most populous states—California, Texas, and Florida—will have the greatest scarcity of physicians by 2030.[14] Rural and underserved urban communities have lacked enough primary care providers to meet the medical demands of their populations for a long time. Now the problem is spreading into the country's more populated areas.[15]

Government central planning of the health care work force has also impacted mental health services. According to a 2022 Harris Poll conducted for the National Council on Mental Wellbeing, approximately 40 percent of Americans who tried to access those services said they could not get mental health services in the past 12 months, particularly services requiring drug-based therapy. Research indicates that growing numbers of patients are seeking treatment for mental illness, yet supply is unable to meet existing needs. The Centers for Disease Control and Prevention estimates that 23.2 percent of adults aged 18–44 received mental health services in 2021, an increase from 18.5 percent in 2019.[16] A 2020 report by the Kaiser Family Foundation concluded that the United States had only enough psychiatrists to meet 26 percent of the population's needs.[17]

Amid these shortages, state licensing and scope of practice laws bar people from seeing numerous health professionals from whom they can receive physical and mental health services.

It is impossible to know what other health profession niches might have already developed for patients to access were it not for the impediments to innovation that licensing and scope of practice laws create.

Following are a few examples of health professions that the government restricts or completely bars patients from patronizing. The list is far from exhaustive.

Advanced Practice Registered Nurses

An advanced practice registered nurse (APRN) is a registered nurse (RN) who has earned a graduate-level degree and has trained in one of the four recognized APRN specialties: nurse practitioner (NP); certified registered nurse anesthetist (CRNA); certified nurse midwife (CNM); and clinical nurse specialist (CNS). NPs provide medical care to patients with or without physician supervision, depending on the state; CRNAs are responsible for administering anesthesia; CNMs specialize in women's reproductive health and childbirth; and CNSs may have a similar role to NPs, but they are typically involved in education, research, and consulting.[18]

The University of Colorado established the first nurse practitioner program in the United States in 1965.[19] Since then, the medical and advanced practice nursing professions have battled in front of state lawmakers over whether the government should allow patients to access primary care services from nurse practitioners. The two professions debate whether NPs provide primary care services that are comparable in quality to that provided by physicians. Both opponents and proponents of expanding nurse practitioners' scope of practice can cite literature comparing care by NPs to care by physicians. Opponents point to the differences in education and training: physicians must complete 10,000 to 16,000 hours of clinical education and training, while NPs only have 500 to 720 hours.[20] Proponents point to health outcomes; they cite research that NPs provide safe, comparable care to their physician counterparts.[21]

Studying and comparing patient outcomes with NPs versus physicians as primary care providers is challenging, however. For example, there's the matter of self-selection bias, where certain patients may prefer physicians. It is difficult to adjust the data based on the complexity of patients' conditions. For example, patients who have comorbidities often see specialists. Studies should also consider cost (NPs cost less compared to managed care systems) and access to primary care. In many states, NPs and physician assistants tend to practice in rural and underserved areas.

Recently, researchers reported on a large quasi-experimental study designed to minimize confounding factors and offer the best comparison of NP to physician-provided care. The study examined differences in clinical outcomes, service utilization, and health care costs between NP-assigned and physician-assigned patients. It used administrative data from the Veterans Health Administration (VHA), one of the largest integrated care systems in the United States.[22]

The VHA reassigned patients whose primary care physician had left the VHA to either another physician or an NP, independent of the patient's health, thus introducing a pseudo-random feature to the study. The final sample included 806,434 patients in 530 VHA facilities across the United States. After comparing patient conditions pre- and post-reassignment and between primary care providers, the study found that NP-assigned patients had similar total costs and similar clinical outcomes to those of physician-assigned patients and were less likely to require hospitalization.[23]

Today, there are more than 365,000 certified nurse practitioners in the United States, nearly three-quarters of whom deliver primary care services.[24] Some states allow patients to seek services from NPs but require the NPs to be either employed and supervised by physicians or to contract with physicians to "collaborate" with them in their otherwise independent practices. States also vary regarding the scope of services they permit patients to seek from NPs. As of March 2023, 27 states had granted "full practice authority" to NPs, meaning that the NPs can practice to the full extent of their training without a supervising or collaborating physician, diagnose, order tests, prescribe medication, and otherwise independently treat patients.[25]

To be sure, NPs don't undergo the years of education and training endured by physicians, particularly ones trained in specialties. But the data on primary care suggest that NPs provide comparable services. Like physicians, NPs are professionals with a professional code of ethics. Like physicians, if NPs encounter a patient with a clinical problem for which they lack expertise, they will consult or refer the patient to a professional with the appropriate knowledge and experience. Some lawmakers might believe people should choose physicians over nurse practitioners for primary care services, but the choice should not be up to lawmakers. The only ones who should make that choice are patients, as autonomous adults.

Certified registered nurse anesthetists are another type of advanced practice registered nurse. Physicians trained nurses to provide anesthesia for their patients beginning in the early 19th century. Alice Magaw, who worked for what is now known as the Mayo Clinic, performed anesthesia research in the early 1800s. Doctor Charles Mayo dubbed her the "Mother of Anesthesia." The first official nurse anesthetist was Sister Mary Bernard, who started providing anesthesia at Saint Vincent Hospital in Erie, Pennsylvania, in 1887.[26] Today, more than 80 percent of rural anesthesia providers are CRNAs.[27]

As a general surgeon, I have worked with CRNAs for years. They have provided excellent anesthesia care to my critically ill and challenging surgical patients. As a professional, when I encounter patients with surgical problems for which I lack expertise, I call in or refer them to surgeons with more knowledge and experience with the problem. CRNAs are bound by their professional ethics to do the same in such situations.

Research shows there is no evidence of any harm to patients when CRNAs work independently of physicians.[28] Yet the Centers for

Medicare and Medicaid Services (CMS) requires CRNAs to report directly to physicians, and it will not pay them for services they provide independently to Medicare and Medicaid patients. The rule reduces the number of well-trained, specialized nurses who are providing anesthesia independently and ties up anesthesiologists who might be otherwise providing care to patients. Fortunately, CMS permits states to opt out of this requirement. To do so, CMS requires governors to send a letter to the agency attesting that they have consulted with the state's boards of medicine and nursing on the access and quality of anesthesia services, that opting out is consistent with state law, and that they have determined it is in the best interest of the citizens of the state to opt out. As of November 2023, 27 states allow patients to access anesthesia services directly from CRNAs.[29]

Physician Assistants

Responding to the need for primary care practitioners, in 1965, Eugene A. Stead, MD, of Duke University Medical Center, established the first program in the country to train physician assistants (PAs), beginning with four navy hospital corpsmen whom he selected for the program. By the 1970s, the profession gained acceptance and support from the medical profession, which viewed PAs not as competitors but as professional adjuncts who must collaborate with and report to supervising physicians.[30] In 1973 in North Carolina, members of the growing profession established the American Academy of Physician Assistants. In 1974, the National Board of Medical Examiners formed the National Commission on Certification of Physician Assistants (NCCPA), which is presently the only organization in the United States that certifies PAs.[31]

Physician assistants must have a bachelor's degree that includes basic science requirements and complete two to three years of classroom and clinical training. They also usually have a master's degree.

Most PAs train further on the job while working with a physician, thus developing expertise in the physician-employer's specialty. PAs can do further study in several postgraduate specialty programs for which the NCCPA offers private, voluntary certification.[32]

All states prohibit patients from choosing services from PAs who are not supervised by physicians to some degree. The supervision requirements and scope of practice restrictions vary by state. They range from limiting PAs to performing limited diagnostic and therapeutic services that a supervising physician expressly delegates (e.g., Florida, Kentucky, Pennsylvania) to practicing independently to the full extent of their training while consulting or collaborating with physicians on an as-needed basis, based on mutually agreed-upon guidelines between the PA and the physician (e.g., North Dakota, Utah, and Wyoming).[33] In most states, the licensing board that regulates physicians also regulates PAs. A handful of states have independent PA licensing boards.

International Medical Graduates

State licensing laws make it very difficult for patients to take advantage of the knowledge and experience of foreign physicians who want to offer their services to people in this country. Furthermore, complex and restrictive immigration regulations make it difficult for foreign-born and educated physicians to work in states independent of state licensing requirements.

A cumbersome approval process that began in the late 1950s places daunting obstacles in the way of international medical graduates (IMGs) who want to practice in the United States, where a regulatory regime keeps a tight rein on the already short supply of doctors.[34] The Educational Commission for Foreign Medical Graduates (ECFMG), a nonprofit organization established in 1956 to "evaluate the readiness" of IMGs to enter American graduate medical education programs (residencies and fellowships), oversees the process.[35] The American

Medical Association and the American Hospital Association recognize the ECFMG as the only standard they will accept for evaluating IMGs who are seeking to offer care in the United States. Both
organizations greatly influence state lawmakers and licensing boards.
(Graduates of Canadian medical schools are not considered IMGs.)
The ECFMG obtained responsibility from the federal government for
visa sponsorship of Exchange Visitor physicians (J-1 visas).

States won't allow patients to seek care from IMGs who received
their diplomas and have been practicing medicine outside of the
United States, often for many years. Before patients may take advantage of their expertise, IMGs must undergo the same process as fresh
US medical school graduates. This means they must pass the ECFMG
certification—including taking and passing all three steps of the US
medical licensing exam—and go through a residency training program again. Then, they must apply for state medical licenses. Many
experienced foreign-trained doctors take positions in ancillary medical fields, such as nurse, lab technician, and radiology technician,
instead of starting all over again. Some enter residency programs in a
specialty completely different than the one they are currently practicing so that they can work as a doctor in this country. Sadly, some even
work in industries or fields where their years of training and experience go unutilized.

The Canadian provinces, Australia at the federal level, and most
European Union (EU) countries have a provisional licensing system
that permits experienced foreign doctors to practice under the supervision of a licensed domestic physician for a designated period. When the
supervisory period is complete, and if the immigrant doctors pass the
same exams that are required of domestic physicians, governments grant
them a permanent license. Governments sometimes require immigrant
doctors to practice for a certain period in an underserved area before
they may practice anywhere in the jurisdiction.[36]

However, despite any reforms that state lawmakers might enact, federal immigration laws remain an obstacle to their smooth implementation. To work in the United States, experienced and licensed physicians in other countries—some of whom may even be on the faculty of foreign medical schools—must win H-1B visas through a lottery and, eventually, obtain permanent residency under the green card caps if they hope to stay here. Congress last updated the low employer-sponsored green card cap in 1990. Special limits on immigrants based on birthplace are causing physicians from India and China, the world's two most populous countries, to face extremely long waits. Many India-born physicians will die waiting for a green card.[37]

In May 2023, Tennessee became the first state to grant provisional licenses to international medical graduates who have full licenses in good standing in other countries and who pass the same standardized medical exams that US medical graduates must pass. After two years of supervision by a Tennessee-licensed physician, they can receive unrestricted licenses.[38] This will give Tennesseans greater choice and access to health care providers. In 2024, several other states enacted reforms like the one Tennessee lawmakers passed, including Florida, Idaho, Iowa, Virginia, and Wisconsin.[39]

Assistant Physicians

Since the early 1950s, hospitals and medical centers that offer postgraduate training (residency) programs have been participating in the National Resident Matching Program (NRMP), which matches graduating medical students with available residency programs.[40] The Association of American Medical Colleges and the National Student Internship Committee created the NRMP to assign graduating medical school students to accredited residency programs.

Applicants communicate directly with the residency programs they are interested in attending. The program directors determine

the applicants' eligibility and may invite them to an interview. The
applicants and program administrators submit lists to the NRMP,
each ranking their preferences. The NRMP then uses a mathemat-
ical algorithm to match the applicants to programs.[41] The NRMP
announces the match results on the Monday of Match Week, which
is the third week of March. The match serves as a binding agreement, signed during the registration process, between the applicant and the program. The NRMP provides a Supplemental Offer
and Acceptance Program for eligible applicants who have not been
matched with any program.[42] This program involves a series of
two-hour-long rounds that include remote interviews conducted
Monday through Thursday of Match Week, during which programs offer available positions to unmatched applicants, both parties rank their preferences, and the NRMP applies the matching
algorithm. Not all programs with open positions choose to partic-
ipate in this, and not all unmatched applicants can find an accredited position.

Unmatched graduates are stuck in limbo, unable to care for patients
and apply the knowledge and clinical skills that they acquired with
their doctorate degrees while also being unable to further hone and
develop those clinical skills with postgraduate training. According
to the American Medical Association, in 2021, roughly 7 percent of
doctor of medicine graduates and 10 percent of doctor of osteopathy
graduates found themselves in that state of limbo.[43]

Some states have reduced the legal barriers that prevent unmatched
medical school graduates from rendering primary care services. In
2014, Missouri became the first state to allow these physicians to
practice as assistant physicians (APs). Not to be confused with PAs,
APs are analogous to an apprenticeship where medical school graduates work for, and collaborate with, licensed primary care physicians
who have clinics in underserved areas of their state. APs, in short, are

apprentice physicians. Such apprenticeships were a common way to train physicians before the modern era of residency programs.[44]

The Missouri program launched in 2017. By February 2023, the addition of APs had increased the state's primary care provider workforce by 3 percent.[45] By the end of 2023, Alabama, Arizona, Arkansas, Idaho, Kansas, Louisiana, Tennessee, and Utah had enacted laws to license APs.

State lawmakers should not prohibit medical school graduates from using their experience as APs as an alternative pathway to unrestricted licensure as physicians. If one or two years of residency plus passing step three of the standardized US medical licensing exam qualifies physicians in most states to practice medicine without board certification as specialists, then three or more years of experience as an AP and passing the same exam should also suffice.[46]

Such an alternative pathway could lead to innovations in how specialty boards certify clinicians. For example, general practice physicians who wish to specialize usually apply to specialty residency training programs. When they complete residency training, they take standardized specialty examinations and seek certification from specialty boards such as the American Board of Internal Medicine, the American Board of Family Medicine, the American Board of Pediatrics, and the American Board of Obstetrics and Gynecology. Thus, increasing the number of nonspecialist general practitioners might incentivize some certifying organizations to develop alternative pathways to certification that place greater emphasis on real-world experience. Certifying organizations might even develop various levels of certification based on applicants' backgrounds and experience.

Without an alternative pathway, state governments will continue to protect the medical profession's virtual monopoly on generating physicians, thus restricting the number of physicians that patients can consult and undermining patients' right to choose their provider.

Prescribing Psychologists

Mental illness is a serious and growing problem in the United States. The National Institute of Mental Health estimates that 52.9 million, or nearly one in five, adults in the United States live with mental illness.[47] In 2021, nearly 48,000 US residents died from suicide.[48] Suicide is the second leading cause of death among people aged 10–34 in the United States.[49] Research indicates that growing numbers of patients are seeking treatment for mental illness, yet supply is unable to meet existing needs.

Clinical psychologists diagnose and treat mental health disorders using various methods of talk therapy. States require clinical psychologists to obtain a doctoral degree in clinical psychology (PhD or PsyD) from a state-approved institution before they let patients seek their help. Satisfying the requirements that states impose to become a clinical psychologist typically takes 8–12 years; many states also require a postdoctoral fellowship, which can add another 1–2 years.[50]

In general, clinical psychologists do not prescribe medications. If they believe that antidepressants, mood stabilizers, or other medications would facilitate therapy, they refer patients to a prescribing practitioner. Usually, the prescribing practitioner of choice is a psychiatrist. Psychiatrists are medical doctors with extensive training in using medication to treat mental illness. Nowadays, psychiatrists function primarily as prescribers. One survey found that only about 10.8 percent of psychiatrists offered any talk therapy.[51] Most engage primarily in pharmacotherapy.

Psychiatrists are costly and in short supply. Initial consultations with a psychiatrist can cost as much as $500 and follow-up visits can range from $100 to $300 per hour.[52] Roughly half of psychiatrists don't accept insurance.[53] Per capita, there are about twice as many clinical psychologists as psychiatrists in the United States (30 versus 16.6 per 100,000 people) and nearly three times as many in rural areas (9.1 versus 3.4 per 100,000 people).[54] Many rural counties lack an adequate number of psychiatrists. Patients must often travel long distances to see psychiatrists to whom their clinical psychologists have referred them.[55]

Clinical psychologists can also refer patients to other prescribing practitioners, including specialists in general surgery, like me, as well as nonspecialist physicians and, where state law permits, physician assistants and nurse practitioners. States allow these clinicians to prescribe antidepressants, mood stabilizers, and antipsychotics even though they often lack expertise in these medications. Referring clinical psychologists often advise and support these practitioners on which drug, or combination of drugs, to prescribe. In some cases, clinical psychologists may have more expertise about these medications than the prescribing practitioners whom they advise.

For example, suppose a clinical psychologist in a remote area needed help getting a patient on medication, and a general surgeon like me was the only licensed prescriber nearby. In that case, the psychologist can ask the general surgeon to prescribe the medication but would likely need to advise the surgeon regarding the dose and possible drug interactions because surgeons lack experience prescribing psychiatric medications.

More than 30 years ago, the US Department of Defense trained doctorate-level clinical psychologists to prescribe psychological medications to increase the workforce of prescribing psychotherapists. The American College of Neuropsychopharmacology reviewed the Department of Defense training program. It concluded, "It seems clear that a two-year program—one year didactic, one-year clinical practicum that includes at least six months of inpatient rotation—can transform licensed clinical psychologists into prescribing psychologists who can function effectively and safely and expand the delivery of mental health treatment to a variety of patients in a cost-effective way."[56] A Government Accountability Office review of the program concurred.[57]

Today, prescribing psychologists (RxPs) who have undergone this additional training practice at several federal agencies—including the military, the US Public Health Service Commissioned Corps, and the Indian Health Service. Those who have obtained similar training and passed the nationally standardized Psychopharmacology Exam for Psychologists (PEP) have been practicing in the territory of Guam (since 1999); New Mexico (2002); Louisiana (2004); Illinois (2014); Iowa (2016); Idaho (2017); Colorado (2023); and Utah (2024).

Often, in states where competent prescribing psychologists seek government permission to offer their services to residents, representatives of the medical and psychiatric professions fiercely oppose them. These incumbents try to convince lawmakers that trained-to-prescribe psychotherapists are not safe or competent enough for the government to allow patients to choose them. They ask the politicians, not the patients, to make that assessment. In the state where I practice general surgery, the Arizona Psychiatric Association has used such arguments to oppose a bill that would grant prescriptive authority to clinical psychologists who have completed extra training in clinical psychopharmacology.[58]

The evidence shows that prescribing psychologists prescribe as safely as, and possibly more conservatively than, psychiatrists. They also tend to continue talk therapy with their patients.[59] Research suggests that states that have granted patients access to more prescribing psychotherapists by letting them consult RxPs had statistically significant drops in suicide rates.[60]

Removing government barriers to patients wishing to consult RxPs will increase the supply of competent mental health prescribers, reduce the costs and inconvenience of mental health care, and respect the right of autonomous adults to choose their mental health providers.

Dental Therapists

According to the latest estimates from the Health Resources and Services Administration, there are roughly 12,000 fewer dentists than necessary to service the US population.[61] Dental schools are not graduating students fast enough to keep up with the rate at which dentists are retiring and the population is growing.[62]

The dental therapist profession developed decades ago in New Zealand and Australia. Dental therapists are mid-level dental professionals analogous to physician assistants in the medical profession. These professionals originally provided dental care to children in schools and later expanded to caring for adults. The governments of Australia and New Zealand require dental therapists to earn a bachelor of oral health degree and to contract with a supervising licensed dentist who must be available for the dental therapist to consult at all times and who performs an annual audit of the dental therapist's charts.[63] Beginning in the 1920s, governments in several countries worldwide began lifting restrictions on their residents' right to choose dental therapists for their care.[64]

Dental therapists can provide routine restorative and preventive care, such as cleanings, fillings, simple extractions, and placing temporary crowns. They have more extensive training than dental hygienists but less training than dentists.[65]

The first government in the United States to allow residents to freely access dental therapists was the Alaska Native Tribal Health Consortium in 2004.[66] Dental therapists must receive at least two years of specialized training that awards an associate degree and also complete 400 hours of a clinical preceptorship, which is an apprenticeship with a dental mentor that culminates in certification. Dental therapists must contract with a supervising dentist but they may practice remotely from any dentist's office. According to a 2017 report, 40,000 people in 81 underserved tribal and rural communities in Alaska had access to dental care because the government did not restrict their ability to consult dental therapists.[67]

Since that time, several other state governments have followed suit, including Arizona, Maine, Michigan, Minnesota, and Washington.[68] Patients in more than 50 countries can also get routine restorative and preventive care from dental therapists.[69]

The American Dental Association endorses the dental therapist profession, and its Commission on Dental Accreditation adopted dental therapy education standards in 2015. Nevertheless, lawmakers considering legislation that would allow dental therapists to practice in their states often receive pushback from state representatives of the dental profession, who claim to be concerned about patient safety. For example, in Arizona, dentists, including one serving in the state legislature at the time, argued that dental therapists are less trained than dentists and therefore the government shouldn't allow patients to see them. As a result, Arizona lawmakers only allowed patients in tribal areas and some remote parts of the state to see dental therapists but deprived other Arizonans of that choice.[70] Similarly, Minnesota's government only allows "low-income, uninsured, and underserved patients," or patients who live in a "dental Health Professional Shortage Area," to access dental therapists.[71]

Licensing and scope of practice laws disrespect patients' autonomy and make it harder for them to get dental care.[72]

Letting Pharmacists Prescribe

As a general surgeon, the most common drugs that I prescribe to patients are pain medications and antibiotics. Frequently I see patients in my office who are on a host of other medications for other conditions. I might not be familiar with some of those medications because they are for conditions that I do not treat in my specialty. When that happens, I phone a local pharmacist and ask if the drug that I am about to prescribe can harmfully interact with any of the patient's other medications and if I need to adjust the dose or prescribe a different drug.

When we doctors treat critically ill surgical patients in intensive care units, we often give them multiple medications at the same time, many of which are administered through complex intravenous infusions. The critical care team makes rounds on those patients at least once daily. All the treatment team members are present to tap into each other's expertise and coordinate therapeutic strategies. The hospital pharmacist is an essential member of the team. We rely on the pharmacist's expertise when we need to adjust, add, or subtract drugs that we are giving patients.

Today, more than half of all licensed pharmacists have doctor of pharmacology degrees (PharmD), for which they receive as much classroom time and nearly as much clinical instruction as medical doctors.[73] All 50 states and the District of Columbia now allow pharmacists to prescribe to some degree.[74] This includes prescribing and performing immunization, HIV pre- and post-exposure prophylaxis, hormonal contraceptives, and smoking cessation products. In Australia, Canada, New Zealand, the United Kingdom, and several major European countries including France, Germany, and Italy, drug regulators have a third alternative to the prescription and nonprescription (over-the-counter, or OTC) drug categories: pharmacist-only or "behind-the-counter." This third category requires patients to speak with a pharmacist before purchasing a drug.[75]

In the United States, despite calls by medical experts to allow women to purchase hormonal contraceptives over the counter, the Food and Drug Administration (FDA) will not permit women to buy them without a permission slip in the form of a prescription from a licensed health care practitioner.[76] To work around this, almost half the states have authorized pharmacists, who fit the FDA's licensed health care practitioner requirement, to prescribe hormonal contraceptives.[77] In 2019, California lawmakers authorized pharmacists to prescribe HIV pre- and post-exposure prophylaxis (PrEP and PEP) to make it easier for people to access those drugs.[78] Since then, nine other state legislatures have followed California's lead.[79] Although states vary in the details, all 50 authorize pharmacists to administer vaccinations.[80]

New Zealand and the United Kingdom have allowed pharmacists with extra training to test patients and prescribe drugs for various health conditions, and Australian lawmakers are considering the same.[81] The Canadian province of Alberta has allowed pharmacists who have been in practice for at least one year to test and treat the most common medical conditions since 2006.[82] Several other provinces, including Ontario, Canada's most populous, have been adopting reforms that mimic Alberta's to varying degrees.[83]

One recent study published in the *Journal of the American Medical Association* found that pharmacists prescribing and dispensing medication to treat high blood pressure resulted in greater patient compliance and was less costly.[84] As professionals, the pharmacists are ethically bound to refer patients who need comprehensive follow-up care to physicians after they prescribe and dispense medication to them to start the treatment.

In 2019, Idaho expanded pharmacists' scope of practice, allowing them to prescribe preventive medication, perform tests, and treat every condition where a new diagnosis is not necessary, as well as most health conditions that are minor and self-limiting, such as urinary tract infections, strep throat, and upper respiratory infections. They can also prescribe hormonal contraceptives and HIV pre- and post-exposure prophylaxis.[85] Since then, lawmakers in Colorado and Montana have similarly expanded pharmacists' scope of practice. In 2020, Florida began permitting pharmacists to test and prescribe medicines for minor and non-chronic health conditions, but only if they contract with a physician who will supervise them in a "collaborative practice arrangement," which can be quite cumbersome.[86] The Florida Medical

Association opposes expanding pharmacists' scope of practice and referred to even this limited expansion as "ill-conceived."[87]

This country has a shortage of physicians and dentists, but pharmacies are abundant. Many are open 24 hours. Many people in remote areas have easier access to a pharmacy than to a primary care clinician. But even people in densely populated areas with easier access to clinicians can save time and money if governments let pharmacists prescribe. Think of the convenience of going to a nearby pharmacy to get treatment for a routine condition without taking time off from work, traveling, and sitting in the waiting room to see a clinician, knowing in advance what the problem is and what the clinician will prescribe.

Expect other prescribing health professionals—including physicians, NPs, and PAs—to push back on the idea. Expect them to tell lawmakers that autonomous adults cannot be trusted to choose correctly between a pharmacist or a clinician for their health concerns. These arguments should not persuade lawmakers who respect patient autonomy.

Bringing Back Autonomy

Ideally, states should repeal all health professional licensing laws. Licensing laws do little to protect the public from poor quality care and serve as barriers to new entrants and innovations in the health care professions. States could accredit third-party certification organizations to perform licensing boards' functions.[88] Such organizations could review the credentials, education, and real-world experience of domestic and international applicants and certify them as competent to provide various health care services. These organizations could provide crucial information to help patients decide which clinician to see and to help hospitals, health care facilities, third-party payers, and liability insurers decide with which clinicians to affiliate.

One proposal would create a voluntary alternative pathway involving third-party certification that could coexist with state licensing schemes and gradually replace them. The proposal calls for private certifying organizations to register with the state to privately certify individuals to practice an occupation or profession if they meet the certifying organizations' criteria. States would allow multiple certifying organizations to vet members of the same occupation or profession, competing to provide consumers with high-quality credentialing services. Such an alternative pathway would complement the existing licensing system.[89]

If repealing licensing laws is not feasible, states should refrain from adding established and rising health care professions or specialties to those requiring state licensure or certification. States should also enact laws recognizing practitioners' licenses from other states. In 2019, Arizona became the first state to enact such a universal licensing law, and several states have since passed different versions of such laws.[90] These laws should not require that practitioners reside in the jurisdiction where they offer their services. This is particularly important for people living in urban areas that stretch across state lines, such as Kansas City, New York City, and Washington, DC. And lawmakers should permit all health professions to practice to the full extent of their training, even when it overlaps the expertise of competing professions. A strong demand for information will ensure that a healthy market of competing entities that monitor and rate the competence and effectiveness of the various professions will develop. Autonomous adults will then use this information when they exercise the right to make their own health care decisions.

CHAPTER 3

Certificate of Need Laws

Consider the following scenario. Two graduates of a culinary arts academy collaborate on a unique set of recipes that fuse elements of Indian and Mexican cuisine. They decide to open a restaurant with décor blending both cultures. They have a pretty good idea of where to locate the restaurant. Before raising capital from investors, they must get approval from the state government's restaurant necessity commission.

The commission comprises representatives of the state's most prominent restaurateurs, the state dietician society, and the state's department of health. They review the new restaurant application and invite the applicants to a hearing. The restaurateurs on the commission don't think the public would be interested in this innovative cuisine, and besides, there are already enough restaurants per capita in the state to meet diners' needs. The representative from the dietician society expresses concern that an Indian/Mexican fusion diet might be too rich in carbohydrates. The department of public health representative sees no problem with the request so long as their health inspectors sign off on it. Unfortunately for the applicants, the commission decides that the public doesn't need another restaurant to choose from, and it is probably not in their best interests to eat this new cuisine.

The entrepreneurs' new restaurant never opens. The public will never know what they are missing.

The above scenario might seem far-fetched. Most people would consider the idea of a restaurant necessity commission ridiculous. Yet certificate of need commissions are the norm for those who want to offer the public new health care facilities or services.

History of Certificate of Need Laws

In 1974, Congress passed the National Health Planning and Resources Development Act, which requires states to implement certificate of need (CON) commissions in order to receive funding through certain federal programs.[1] Certificate of need laws require entities that seek to open new hospitals or health facilities or to add beds or equipment to existing ones to get permission from a certificate of need commission, which then decides if the public needs them. Autonomous adults don't get to decide if they need—or want to be able to choose—any additional providers. The government does that for them.

In 1986, Congress repealed the requirement that states enact CON laws. By 1990, 11 states—California, Colorado, Idaho, Kansas, Minnesota, New Mexico, South Dakota, Texas, Utah, Wisconsin, and Wyoming—had repealed their CON laws. Arizona repealed all its CON laws except for one—it still requires ambulance services to obtain a certificate of need. By 2023, 35 states and the District of Columbia still required some or most health care providers to obtain certificates of need in order to open new facilities or to expand or add equipment to existing ones.[2]

Certificate of need laws are a classic example of central planning. They would be more aptly named "permission slips to compete." As with the hypothetical restaurant example, incumbent providers heavily influence CON commissions. Lawmakers attempting to reform or repeal CON laws often meet fierce resistance from the incumbents, who claim they only have the interests of the public in mind.

Policymakers in the Nixon administration promoted certificate of need laws based on the theory that restricting the supply of health care services would somehow reduce demand for those services and thus restrain health care spending. However, they didn't consider that private or government-run third-party payers pay for most health care services. This insulates most patients from the prices of these services, while the third-party payers absorb the costs. Health care consumers with little skin in the game have no incentive to shop for cost-effective services. When price signals can't operate, demand continues to rise despite a restricted supply. Shortages inevitably develop while prices paid by third-party payers increase at a greater rate than would have otherwise occurred. This is basic economics.

The only way to reduce health care expenditures when third-party payers largely insulate health care consumers from price signals is to decrease availability and access to health care. In a George Mason University Mercatus Center working paper, a review of 20 academic studies found that CON laws largely failed to achieve their goal of reducing health care costs and concluded that the overwhelming evidence shows that CON laws are associated with higher per unit costs and higher expenditures.[3] The numbers speak for themselves: national per capita health expenditures increased from $2,354 in 1974 to $12,914 in 2021 (in constant 2021 US dollars).[4]

Despite CON laws' ineffectiveness, most states still have a variety of them on the books—and the entrenched incumbents want to keep it that way. The various state laws differ in the type and number of restricted facilities and expenditures. For example, Ohio restricts only long-term care services, while Kentucky restricts 18 different types of health care facilities.[5]

Protecting Hospitals, Not Patients

The certificate-granting process effectively gives monopoly privileges to existing hospitals and facilities. When new providers petition for a certificate, the commissions usually permit established providers to testify against their would-be competitors.[6] This means that some health care facilities can openly challenge the right to exist of any new facility that might hurt their bottom line.

Indeed, hospital administrators openly admit that protection against competition, thanks to CON laws, has become an integral part of their business model. Hospital administrators argue against repealing CON laws, claiming that these laws let them generate enough revenue to provide 24-hour emergency services and uncompensated care. Lobbyists representing rural hospitals successfully prevented lawmakers from repealing Kentucky's CON laws in 2024, persuading them that repeal might result in new competitors drawing more lucrative non-Medicaid patients away from hospitals that have a high proportion of Medicaid patients, thus endangering their ability to maintain all their services.[7] However, physicians and other health care practitioners also provide uncompensated care and other services. Yet state professional organizations don't argue for creating a certificate of need requirement before allowing additional doctors, nurses, psychologists, physical therapists, and other types of health care practitioners to set up practices in their state. And the public would justifiably deride the organizations if they did.

New health care professionals entering a state may provide competition to incumbents. This has not stunted the growth of the health care professions. Rather, it has benefited health care consumers by increasing choice and access.

According to one health care publication, "Hospitals tend to view CON restrictions favorably when they serve to exclude [competing] facilities from entering a market but may take steps to circumvent the CON application process where their own expansion is concerned."[8]

The 1974 National Health Planning and Resources Development Act explicitly stated that one goal of CON laws was to encourage hospital substitutes, such as ambulatory surgery centers.[9] Yet ironically, 23 states now restrict ambulatory surgery centers, which are common hospital substitutes that compete with traditional hospitals.[10]

Both nursing homes and home health care services provide long-term care and hospice care. Many states that have repealed some CON laws retain them for nursing homes. Comparisons between states with some CON laws and those with no CON laws show that nursing homes—rather than alternatives like home health care—dominate hospice expenditures in states with CON laws.[11] A 2021 Morning Consult poll found an overwhelming majority of adults prefer home health care to nursing home care.[12]

A 2016 Mercatus Center working paper concluded, "The presence of a CON program is associated with 30 percent fewer total hospitals per 100,000 state population and 30 percent fewer rural hospitals per 100,000 rural population."[13] A 2020 Mercatus Center working paper found that states with CON laws spend more per patient on Medicare and Medicaid in rural areas. Per patient hospital readmission rates, ambulance utilization rates, and emergency department utilization rates are also higher in rural areas of states that have CON laws.[14]

Birthing centers have been gaining popularity as alternative venues for labor and delivery. Nurse midwives usually operate them. In some regions of the country, particularly rural areas, birthing centers enable women to give birth in culturally familiar places in a more comforting environment than they would find in a hospital.[15] An added benefit of birthing centers is that they provide additional options for mothers in labor in rural areas, who must often travel very long distances to deliver at a hospital. Freestanding birthing centers take only low-risk patients. The evidence to date suggests that freestanding birthing centers are associated with lower preterm delivery rates, higher birth weights, higher breastfeeding rates, and lower rates of Caesarean sections.[16] Certificate of need laws are associated with fewer birthing centers in a state, yet currently, 14 states require birthing centers to obtain a certificate of need.[17]

Women have been giving birth to babies in their homes since the beginning of recorded history, and in modern times they are increasingly opting for home births.[18] Fortunately, they don't need to obtain a certificate of need from the government before having their baby at home.

Ambulance Services

Then there is the growing problem of "ambulance deserts."[19] In many parts of the United States, ambulance services are so scarce that people may need to wait an hour or longer for an ambulance to arrive. According to a recent study by the University of Southern Maine, 4.5 million Americans live in ambulance deserts, of whom 2.3 million live in rural counties. The researchers defined an ambulance desert as "a populated census block with its geographic center outside of a 25-minute ambulance service area."[20]

The study found that roughly 80 percent of counties in the United States have ambulance deserts, but that ambulance deserts were much more common in rural counties than in urban ones. The counties with the highest share of ambulance deserts were in the Appalachian regions of the South.[21]

A 2023 *Wall Street Journal* article reported that more than 55 ambulance services had closed nationwide since 2021. In many cases they had difficulty hiring people who were willing to train for this high-pressure job at their own expense. Adding to the problem is the fact that the ambulance business can often be unprofitable. For example, service providers in rural areas make fewer calls per year than in urban areas, often traveling longer distances with higher fuel costs.[22] There is no simple fix to the country's ambulance desert problem. Its causes are multifaceted. But while state CON laws are not responsible for this problem, they do play a role.[23]

States Admit the Problem

During the COVID-19 pandemic, many states realized that their CON laws left them unprepared for the sudden surge in demand for critical care and other health care services and they were straitjacketed by bureaucratic red tape. Twenty states suspended their CON laws and four other states issued emergency certificates of need—thereby bypassing the usually months-long certificate application process.[24] This was a tacit admission that certificate of need laws impede the rapid response of the health care system to sudden changes.

We have seen—and continue to see—countries that embrace central planning fall victim to what economists call "the knowledge problem." It is impossible to predict how many intensive care unit beds, general beds, or other health care facilities and services will be necessary to serve a growing and dynamic population. Markets are the most accurate and efficient way of allocating goods and services. Yet they are not allowed to properly function in America's critical health care sector.

Christina Sandefur of the Goldwater Institute characterizes CON laws as a "competitor's veto."[25] But CON laws are even more nefarious. These laws assault patient autonomy by empowering a government commission and its cronies to decide how many and what kinds of health care services adults may seek. States should repeal all certificate of need laws.

CHAPTER 4

End the Food and Drug Administration's Power to Require Prescriptions

The Right to Contraception

Women in more than 100 countries can get birth control pills over the counter.[1] Yet the US government requires women to ask other adults for permission slips, in the form of a prescription, before getting access to hormonal contraceptives.

Tens of millions of American women—more than four out of five women who have had sexual intercourse—have used oral contraceptives, which are crucial for reducing unwanted pregnancies and the incidence of abortion.[2] Obtaining a physician's prescription can add up to $200 plus time and inconvenience to the cost of "the pill."[3] Nearly a third of American women who seek prescriptions for oral contraceptives report having difficulty obtaining them, citing nonmonetary obstacles, such as getting to their doctors' appointments, twice as often as they cite the difficulty of paying for the appointments.[4]

The Institute for Women's Policy Research recommended in 2000 that the FDA let women obtain birth control pills over the counter.[5] The American College of Obstetrics and Gynecology has called on the FDA to remove the prescription requirement on all hormonal contraceptives since the early 2000s. In 2019, the college reiterated its call, adding that women of all ages should have over-the-counter access to hormonal contraceptives.[6] It's notable for the college to take that position, considering that ob-gyn doctors are paid to prescribe hormonal contraceptives. The American Academy of Family Physicians and the American Medical Association have long echoed the American College of Obstetrics and Gynecology's position.[7]

After medical experts had been clamoring for years, the FDA finally announced in mid-2023 that it would permit women to obtain one brand (Opill) of one form of oral contraceptive without a prescription: the so-called mini-pill, a progestin-only pill, which is not as easy to use as combination oral contraceptives. [8]

Unlike regular birth control pills, which contain two female hormones, estrogen and progesterone, the mini-pill doesn't affect milk production in nursing mothers and is less likely to cause blood clots in women who smoke. But, to add perspective, pregnancy is much more likely to cause clots than any pill designed to prevent it. And while the mini-pill may be slightly safer than combination birth control pills, it has significant drawbacks.[9] For example, women must take the mini-pill at the same hour each day. If they take it three hours late, they must use another form of contraception for the rest of the month and start the cycle again.[10] It's the same if they miss a day. With regular (combination) birth control pills, if women miss a day in the cycle, they can take two pills the next day.

Alas, the FDA doesn't trust women to use combination pills correctly or to seek advice from experts. This is nothing new. It took years of prodding and a federal court order to get the FDA to allow women of all ages to obtain emergency contraception—the so-called morning-after pill. One famous brand is Plan B.[11] The FDA started permitting women to buy emergency contraceptives with a prescription in 1999. Shortly after that, various medical experts, women's advocacy groups, and even FDA advisory panels urged the agency to let women of all ages obtain them without a prescription. Finally, in 2013, a federal court ordered the FDA to let women of all ages obtain emergency contraception over the counter.[12] Today, people can get emergency contraceptives in vending machines.[13] It's a sad irony that the government lets women get Plan B over the counter but doesn't let them get what many women might call "Plan A."

Naloxone, the Overdose Cure

The FDA does not limit its paternalism to women. For years, experts have called on the agency to let people obtain naloxone, the opioid overdose antidote, without a prescription. Residents of Italy have been able to buy naloxone over the counter for more than 20 years, and Australians have been doing so since 2016.[14]

The FDA has allowed clinicians to prescribe naloxone since 1971. The drug works by blocking opioid receptors. It is an effective remedy that laypeople can safely administer with minimal training, using either a nasal spray or an intramuscular auto-injector. The FDA, aware of the drug's safety profile, began in 2016 to directly and indirectly ask the makers of naloxone nasal spray to request that the agency remove the prescription requirement. The agency can make the switch without the manufacturer requesting it. However, the agency deferred to the drugmaker, who lacked the financial incentive to market naloxone over the counter. (Third-party payers rarely pay for over-the-counter drugs, and the makers of naloxone were charging them higher prices than they would be able to get for the drug in an over-the-counter market.)[15]

Most states have developed workarounds to make it easier for opioid users and people close to them to obtain naloxone. That usually involves authorizing pharmacists to prescribe the drug or letting licensed clinicians issue a standing order that lets pharmacists distribute it without a patient-specific prescription.[16] Finally, in early 2023, the

FDA removed the prescription requirement for naloxone nasal spray.[17] Injectable naloxone still requires a prescription.

Many substance-use harm-reduction organizations operating on tight budgets still ask community physicians to issue standing orders that enable them to purchase prescription-only injectable naloxone, which is much cheaper than the nasal spray version.[18] I issue standing orders for injectable naloxone to assist a prominent harm-reduction organization in my home state of Arizona.

These stories are just a few examples of the many ways in which the government, out of paternalistic precaution or for political reasons, blocks adults from exercising their right to self-medicate by requiring them to get prescriptions in order to use certain drugs.

Federal law grants the FDA the power to prevent competent adults from accessing certain drugs unless they spend the time and money required to get a prescription. This practice started when the FDA interpreted the Food, Drug, and Cosmetic Act of 1938 (FDCA) as granting it this power, even though the bill's sponsors disavowed any such desire.[19] Congress made the agency's interpretation official when it codified this usurped power with the 1951 Durham-Humphrey Amendment to the FDCA.[20]

It wasn't always this way. Before 1938, federal legislation typically respected the right of individuals to self-medicate.[21] Aside from specific instances such as the Harrison Narcotics Act of 1914, which mandated prescriptions for narcotics surpassing established limits, there were no overarching federal mandates requiring consumers to secure a physician's prescription before obtaining a medication. As former FDA general counsel Peter Barton Hutt noted in 1982, determining whether a patient needed a physician's permission to purchase a drug was entirely at the manufacturer's discretion.[22] It was common practice for drug manufacturers to market certain products as being intended for use under a physician's supervision and sometimes requiring a physician's prescription.

Unless that was the case, adults were free to purchase any nonnarcotic drug for self-medication without a doctor's prescription.

Most patients sought the advice of medical professionals before purchasing drugs at pharmacies, although the law didn't require them to do so. Economist Sam Peltzman reported that, by 1938, "about one-third of drug purchases were being made under a doctor's prescription."[23] Adults considered the guidance their physicians provided in conjunction with other sources of information, such as the perspectives and recommendations offered by pharmacists. But ultimately, consumers independently decided which advice to follow and which medications to use.

The private sector provided consumers and their physicians with resources to make informed decisions. In 1820, collaborative efforts among physicians, pharmacists, and pharmacy schools led to the establishment of the United States Pharmacopeial Convention—a private, nonprofit organization dedicated to disseminating pharmaceutical information. This organization continues its commitment by regularly publishing and updating the United States Pharmacopeia (USP), a respected compendium encompassing drugs and their uses, which covers indications, dosage recommendations, warnings, contraindications, and off-label uses. Additionally, the organization produces the National Formulary, which includes information on drugs, dietary supplements, vitamins, and minerals. The National Formulary sets standards for composition, purity, strength, storage, and labeling, and defines analytical tests and methods to ensure adherence to these standards.[24]

The Pure Food and Drug Act

When the federal government began regulating pharmaceuticals in the early 20th century, it continued to respect the right to self-medicate. Reacting to highly publicized instances of drug manufacturers defrauding, misleading, or even harming consumers, Congress passed the Pure Food and Drug Act (PFDA) of 1906. Rather than infringe on the right to self-medicate or limit medical autonomy, the act attempted to provide more information to consumers and physicians. The PFDA—in a case of the law catching up to reality—codified the privately created USP and defined a drug as "adulterated" if it failed to meet the USP's standards. Those provisions seemed to have little practical effect, since the USP was already the widely recognized standard of practice. The PFDA also defined the crime of "misbranding," stating that a drugmaker misbranded a drug if it contained alcohol, opium, cocaine, or any other dangerous or potentially addictive substance and failed to list those ingredients, and their proportional inclusion, on the product label. The US Bureau of Chemistry, which implemented the new law, had no authority to determine the efficacy of pharmaceuticals.[25] In 1927, Congress reorganized the Bureau of Chemistry into the Food, Drug, and Insecticide Administration. In 1930, Congress renamed the agency the Food and Drug Administration.

Things dramatically changed in 1938 when Congress saw the need to respond to a highly publicized tragedy. The S. E. Massengill Company had been successfully marketing a safe and effective new antimicrobial drug called sulfanilamide. Sulfanilamide, a so-called sulfa drug, was the first effective antimicrobial, becoming available to the public roughly a decade before penicillin. The company decided to release a sweet-flavored liquid "elixir" formulation to make the drug easier for children and others to ingest. It produced the sulfa drug according to specifications, but its solvent did not meet the USP standard for branding as an elixir. The USP, and therefore the PFDA, allowed only solutions that used alcohol as the solvent to bear the name "elixir." Rather than use alcohol, the company used diethylene glycol—a close chemical cousin of antifreeze (ethylene glycol). The solution poisoned hundreds of consumers, causing extremely painful reactions and 105 deaths, including 34 children.[26]

Massengill recalled the product. The government fined the company the highest legally allowed fine for mislabeling its product. Had the company called the product a "solution" rather than an "elixir," the company would not have violated any law. The company settled several lawsuits with the families of the victims.[27] Massengill ultimately filed for bankruptcy and the chemist who created the formula committed suicide.[28]

In response to this tragedy, Congress passed the Food, Drug, and Cosmetic Act. One of its key provisions required manufacturers to file a new drug application with the FDA before marketing any new drug. The application had to include information on the drug's composition, safety test results, and the manufacturer's quality controls. If the FDA approved the drug as safe, or failed to act on it within 60 days, the manufacturer could proceed to market. (The act allowed existing drugs with a proven safety record to remain on the market. This is why regular and neutral protamine Hagedorn (NPH) insulin, developed decades earlier, are still available in the United States without a prescription.) The FDCA also imposed stricter misbranding rules. It required manufacturers to list all ingredients in their precise amounts on labels. Crucially, the new law made manufacturers provide detailed instructions on their labels that were understandable to people with a rudimentary education. The FDCA waived the labeling requirement if the drugmaker decided to require a physician's prescription before manufacturers could sell it to the public.

However, the act didn't explicitly require manufacturers to designate any drugs as prescription-only.[29] In fact, even as Congress debated and enacted the FDCA, its supporters paid homage to the right to self-medicate. Supporters argued that the act was merely a truth-in-labeling bill that sought to make self-medication safer by furnishing consumers with more information. Testifying before Congress in support of an early iteration of the law, FDA director

Walter G. Campbell repeatedly avowed that the bill's purpose and effect would be to facilitate self-medication, not restrict it. The House committee that reported the bill in 1938 wrote: "The bill is not intended to restrict in any way the availability of drugs for self-medication. On the contrary, it is intended to make self-medication safer and more effective."[30]

And this made sense. A government-imposed prescription requirement would not have prevented the tragedy; of the 105 consumers who died, 100 took the drug under the direction of government-licensed physicians.[31] If anything, the elixir sulfanilamide tragedy provided evidence that, even in the absence of government-imposed prescription requirements, consumers overwhelmingly seek advice from trusted experts before taking medications—even if those experts sometimes do not deserve their patients' trust. In this case, those experts had government licenses to practice medicine. As I explained in chapter 3, a license to practice medicine does not protect the public from a doctor's poor judgment. Many patients often hesitate to ask doctors important questions regarding the risks and benefits of the medicines they are prescribing, and instead defer to their status as experts.[32]

The FDCA's costly labeling requirement, along with an exemption for prescription-only drugs, transformed a law that purported to facilitate self-medication into a sweeping curtailment of the right to self-medicate. The expense and liability associated with compliance with the labeling requirement effectively coerced manufacturers into selling many drugs as prescription-only. Commercial advantage and risk aversion pushed in the same direction. Classifying or reclassifying drugs as prescription-only was likely attractive to drug manufacturers because it allowed them to charge higher prices, sidestep extremely costly labeling requirements, and avoid enforcement actions by the FDA.

As regulators implemented the FDCA, they quickly deviated from its authors' stated goal of promoting informed self-medication and began interpreting the law as empowering the agency to require prescriptions. As economic historian Peter Temin explains:

> By the end of 1938, the FDA had announced that the government would sharply curtail this freedom of choice. Consumers, the FDA said, were not competent to make their own drug choices. . . . The government had delegated the consumers' choice to manufacturers and doctors—and nobody commented.
>
> . . .
>
> This change in the underlying assumptions of drug legislation came about through internal FDA processes. The shift from assuming a capable consumer to assuming an incompetent consumer was made within the FDA within six months of the Federal Food, Drug, and Cosmetics Act's passage. Not only was the shift in assumptions not controversial, the method by which it was accomplished occasioned no comment as well. The decisions of the FDA were ratified by the courts and enacted into statute by the Congress. Neither branch of the government undertook to question the FDA's assumptions.[33]

Statutory respect for patient autonomy came to a complete end when Congress codified the FDA's ostensible usurpation of the right to self-medicate by passing the Durham-Humphrey Amendment to the FDCA in 1951. This amendment officially empowered the FDA to require patients to obtain a physician's permission before purchasing certain drugs. It prohibits dispensing a prescription-only drug unless the consumer presents a prescription from a government-licensed health care practitioner.

Durham-Humphrey undermines the law's respect for the right to self-medicate. At the same time, it increases the cost of obtaining medications by requiring visits to doctors' offices and pharmacies and may contribute to higher drug prices. It also makes patients less safe.

Self-Medication and Due Diligence

Evidence shows that patients tend to trust prescriptions from expert professionals and don't perform anything resembling the due diligence they perform when purchasing OTC medicines on their own.[34] As a practicing surgeon, I frequently see patients who can't tell me the names of the routine drugs their doctors prescribe to them—or the reasons they take them.

For instance, a study from 2006 in Seattle showed that women were more conservative and cautious in their self-screening for the safe use of oral contraceptives compared to ob-gyn specialists.[35] Meanwhile, doctors prescribed sulfanilamide for infections to 95 percent of patients and supervised their use of the drug. Many of these doctors prescribed it for conditions it was not suited to treat, such as kidney inflammation. Similarly, government-licensed physicians gave thalidomide, which caused birth defects in other countries, to 624 pregnant women during the 1950s and 1960s without disclosing its experimental status.[36]

Medical historian Harry Marks suggests that when the FDA asserted its authority to require prescriptions for certain drugs, it not only removed those drugs from the consumers' reach but intentionally denied consumers information about those drugs. To ensure that prescription-only drugs would only make their way to consumers through physicians, "the FDA would instruct firms to remove from their labels any remaining information that might guide lay users of prescription drugs."[37] Marks argues that these regulations are "best understood as an FDA effort to limit industry abuses of the prescription labeling system."[38]

Economist Sam Peltzman found that enforcement of prescription regulation increased per capita consumption of medicines that tend to be more potent than over-the-counter meds, and suggested there is a moral hazard in shifting consumption toward riskier drugs. He noted a higher rate of drug poisoning in the United States compared to countries that didn't enforce prescription requirements.[39] Peltzman also found deaths from accidental or suicidal poisonings increased by 50 to 100 percent when the FDA began imposing prescription requirements.[40]

Government Control Invites Special-Interest Pleading

When the government controls which drugs are prescription-only, lobbying by special interests influences policy. For example, the FDA approved the nonsedating antihistamine Claritin as a prescription-only drug in 1993. Its manufacturer, Schering-Plough, lobbied successfully for several years to sell it over the counter to patients in Europe while simultaneously making the opposite argument to the FDA. It wasn't until the drug's patent expired in 2002 that the company changed its position, after which the FDA allowed Americans to buy it without a prescription.[41] Before then, American patients only had OTC access to sedating antihistamines, such as Benadryl, which are more dangerous. For example, the Federal Aviation Administration does not permit pilots to fly commercial airlines while taking sedating antihistamines.[42]

Political considerations can also influence the government's control over prescription requirements. They undoubtedly played a role in the FDA's 12-year delay before allowing people to purchase emergency contraceptives without a prescription and its continued foot-dragging regarding OTC hormonal contraceptives, despite medical experts repeatedly calling on the agency to remove prescription requirements.

The government's control over prescription requirements also contributes to higher drug prices. Prescription drugs tend to bring greater profits because insurance tends to cover them, so drugmakers can charge higher prices to third-party payers. Drug prices usually drop after the FDA reclassifies them as over the counter and they become subject to comparison shopping and closer consumer scrutiny.[43]

A Pathway to Autonomy

To help expand access to pharmaceuticals and restore the right to self-medicate, Congress should strip the FDA of any power to impose prescription requirements. This requires repealing the Durham-Humphrey Amendment and prohibiting the FDA from using other provisions of the Food, Drug, and Cosmetics Act of 1938 to impose prescription requirements, as the agency did between 1938 and 1951. State legislatures could restrict medication access by minors and the cognitively disabled and, if necessary, enact specific limitations on access to certain antibiotics.[44]

As the pharmaceutical industry has developed increasingly complex and sophisticated drugs, including new forms of chemotherapy and immunotherapy, not much would change if Congress passed these reforms. The complexity, sophistication, and risks posed by many modern pharmaceuticals and the threat of tort liability would lead manufacturers to continue to market many drugs as prescription-only. Manufacturers might want to continue requiring prescriptions for drugs that can affect third parties, such as antibiotics—which, if overused, can enable antibiotic-resistant organisms to emerge—and for particularly dangerous drugs, such as narcotics and tranquilizers.

Like they do today, people will continue to consult experts before buying and consuming medications. Those experts include more than members of the medical and dental professions: they can and should consist of nurse practitioners, physician assistants, prescribing psychologists, dental therapists, and pharmacists.

What would change is that patients will have broader access to drugs that are less complex, have established safety records, and are available without a prescription in several other countries. Such drugs include insulin, hormonal contraceptives, injectable naloxone, asthma inhalers, statin drugs, nitroglycerine (for chest pain), and sumatriptan (for migraines).[45]

Removing unnecessary prescription requirements would unburden consumers of the unnecessary time and financial costs of visiting a doctor to obtain a prescription and waiting for a pharmacist to fill it. Consumers would also have many convenient options for purchasing OTC medications, including online services, convenience stores, airport newsstands, grocery stores, vending machines, and more. Low-income people who struggle to pay medical bills and who might otherwise forgo necessary treatment would clearly benefit the most from a reduction in drug prices.

It is impossible to predict which drugs that currently require prescriptions will become available over the counter. However, it is plausible that elementary and secondary schools would more easily stock asthma medications and epinephrine injectors. People with diabetes would likely be able to purchase insulin in bulk via online retailers such as Amazon. Naloxone auto-inject pens could become more widely available at vending machines and in first-aid kits. Places that opioid users frequent might make naloxone available for emergency use, just as many establishments make defibrillators available.

Ending the government's power to require prescriptions would likely reduce drug prices while saving consumers money on medical expenditures. Sam Peltzman writes that removing prescription requirements would trigger price competition among a host of drugs as price-sensitive consumers would comparison shop. He notes:

> The effect on prices is also clear: every study of the matter shows substantial price reductions when drugs move to OTC. Of course, total cost—including the cost of physician visits and the value of the time and trouble of securing prescriptions—declines even further when the drug moves to OTC.[46]

There are intermediate steps that federal and state lawmakers can take toward restoring patient autonomy.[47]

Another option Peltzman suggests is for Congress to periodically remove prescription requirements by giving doctors and patients greater say over whether a drug is safe enough to sell over the counter:

> I suggest the FDA should periodically review existing drugs for eligibility for OTC sales. I further suggest that when any prescription drug passes certain milestones—x million prescriptions sold over y years with a risk profile similar to, say, ibuprofen or aspirin—there should be a rebuttable presumption that the drug becomes OTC-eligible. It would then be up to the drug's producer or producers to take advantage of the opportunity.[48]

This way, the burden of proof to demonstrate why a drug should remain prescription-only would shift to the FDA. This reform would still leave the FDA infringing on individuals' right to self-medicate, but to a lesser extent than it does now.

As a more modest step, Congress could create a new category called "behind the counter." This category, which exists in several other countries, allows consumers to access a drug without a government-mandated prescription.[49] Instead, a pharmacist acts as an intermediary, ostensibly to screen patients to see if the medicine they want is right for them. Manufacturers can seek behind-the-counter status when submitting new drug applications to the FDA. Peltzman's proposal can also apply here: drugs can automatically move to a less restrictive category when they meet specific criteria. Establishing such a third category would not fully restore patients' right to self-medicate but it would reduce the number of unnecessary doctor visits and associated costs.

State lawmakers can help improve patients' choices and access and reduce their health care expenditures as well. States can expand the scope of practice of licensed health professionals to the full extent of their training. By allowing psychologists, dental therapists, and pharmacists to prescribe medications, for example, states can expand health care access while reducing unnecessary costs in time and money.

Reform won't be achieved easily. Special interests in and out of government will mount well-funded resistance. Manufacturers who classify drugs as prescription-only and set prescription prices might perceive threats from competitors offering comparable drugs over the counter to value-conscious consumers. Health professionals may see increased patient access to over-the-counter drugs as a way to reduce the number of in-office appointments. Enabling more self-medication would also loosen the medical professions' hold over adults' medical decisions. However, the most resistant special interest might be the government itself, as Congress and the FDA claim it would be unwise and unsafe to strip them of their authority to make medical decisions for others.[50]

Restoring patient autonomy and the right to self-medicate will be a challenging task. Like most precious things, it requires perseverance and commitment. Like all precious things, it is worth the effort.

CHAPTER 5

End the Government's Drug Approval Monopoly

When Congress enacted the Food Drug and Cosmetic Act (FDCA) in 1938, it gave the federal government monopoly control over the drug approval process. Henceforth, the Food and Drug Administration would not allow any pharmaceutical manufacturer to bring a drug to market unless it determined that the drug was safe. Before the government created this coercive monopoly, private-sector organizations performed that function. The government takeover largely crowded them out or rendered them redundant. One crucial difference between government and private-sector drug certification is that private certification organizations provide consumers with information that they need to make educated treatment decisions but cannot deny them access to medical care.

In the years following enactment of the FDCA, and later, after passage of the Durham-Humphrey Amendment in 1951, Congress continued to increase federal regulation of pharmaceuticals. Among the most significant changes were the Kefauver-Harris Amendments of 1962, which like the FDCA, were a response to a tragedy involving unsafe drugs. In 1998 and 2006, respectively, the FDA approved the drug thalidomide to treat leprosy and multiple myeloma. The drug's adverse side effects, however, include severe and often fatal birth defects when pregnant women take it. When manufacturers marketed thalidomide as a sedative to pregnant women in the late 1950s and early 1960s, it led to an estimated 10,000 cases of fetal abnormalities across 46 countries.[1]

Thalidomide affected relatively few Americans because the FDA, citing safety concerns, refused to approve the drug. However, posing as part of a new drug inquiry, the Merrell Pharmaceutical Company successfully distributed more than 2.5 million thalidomide tablets to 1,270 physicians in the United States for research purposes. Then, those government-licensed physicians prescribed the drug to 20,771 patients, including 3,879 women of childbearing age, 624 of whom were pregnant. These physicians apparently did not tell their patients that the drug was experimental or that the FDA had not approved it. Sadly, 17 children were born in America with thalidomide-associated deformities.[2]

Reacting to the horrifying news and images, Congress passed the Kefauver-Harris Amendments to the FDCA in 1962. The amendments required drug companies to conduct additional tests and trials to demonstrate that new drugs are safe. But, for the first time, Congress also required manufacturers to establish, to the FDA's satisfaction, on a case-by-case basis, that a new drug is *effective* at treating a specific condition. As the FDA notes in its Guidance for Industry, the amendments require "that informed consent be obtained from all research study subjects so that patients would have to be specifically informed if a drug they were being given or prescribed was 'experimental,' something that had not happened in the case of thalidomide."[3]

One may wonder why Congress granted the FDA authority to determine a drug's efficacy before it would allow patients to use it. After all, thalidomide is effective as a sedative—and in treating nausea associated with pregnancy, for that matter. The issue with thalidomide was safety, and the FDA already had sufficient authority to keep it off the market until it was proven safe, as the agency's handling of the drug demonstrates.

What adds an intriguing aspect to the proof-of-efficacy requirement is that Congress, in response to misconduct by pharmaceutical companies and doctors, opted to further restrict patients' autonomy in self-medication. The Durham-Humphrey Amendment hinders consumers' freedom to self-medicate, necessitating getting permission from a government-designated authority before they can purchase specific drugs. Similarly, the Kefauver-Harris Amendments impede consumers' freedom to self-medicate by prolonging the time it takes for them to either exercise this right (in the context of over-the-counter drugs) or obtain medication with a physician's approval (in the case of prescription drugs).

Private testing and safety and efficacy certification predate the FDA and have always existed alongside it. Organizations such as the US Pharmacopeial Convention, the American Medical Association, *Consumer Reports*, medical journals, health insurance plans, foreign regulatory bodies, and others have offered or continue to offer alternative safety and efficacy certification. In 1905, the AMA established its Council on Pharmacy and Chemistry, which charged drug companies to test their products for safety. If products received the AMA Seal of Acceptance, the AMA would allow those products to be advertised in the organization's publications, such as the influential *Journal of the American Medical Association*. As physicians began prescribing or recommending AMA-approved drugs, the council would perform follow-up safety studies and provide information on drugs' efficacy. Preempted by the FDA, however, the AMA ended the program in 1955 but maintains a registry for reporting adverse drug reactions.[4] To this day, *Consumer Reports* evaluates medications, including those that doctors prescribe for patients to use off-label, for price, safety, and efficacy.[5]

Many people cannot imagine a world in which the FDA doesn't have a monopoly on the drug approval process. Yet the FDA does not hold a monopoly in determining the effectiveness of drugs for various purposes. Using a drug for a purpose that the FDA does not officially approve of is termed "off-label use," as the FDA has not yet authorized such usage to be stated on the drug's label. When it comes to utilizing drugs for off-label purposes, endorsements of efficacy originate from entities distinct from the FDA. In addition to *Consumer Reports*, these include other regulatory agencies, health insurers, peer-reviewed medical journals, the US Pharmacopeia, and several other private compendia.[6] When the FDA approves drugs to address specific conditions, manufacturers can only include those approved indications on the drug's label. However, once a drug enters the market, consumers and practitioners can use it for purposes not sanctioned by the FDA, which includes treating different conditions. Similar to how the government grants physicians the freedom to prescribe prescription-only medications for off-label uses, it grants patients the freedom to use over-the-counter drugs for off-label purposes.

Off-label drug uses are common. An estimated 21 percent of prescriptions in the United States are off-label, with the share rising as high as 83 percent for individual drugs.[7] Sometimes off-label drug use yields benefits. For example, clinical researchers found that the anti-nausea medicine thalidomide, which caused birth defects when pregnant women used it for "morning sickness," is effective in treating leprosy and multiple myeloma after clinicians prescribed it off-label. Similarly, doctors recommended aspirin off-label to prevent cardiovascular problems. On the other hand, clinicians can discover that off-label use of a drug can be harmful or inappropriate. For example, some of the deaths from elixir sulfanilamide in 1937 occurred when doctors prescribed it for off-label uses, including to treat kidney inflammation, mercury poisoning, renal colic, and backache.[8]

Off-label drug use is controversial because it is based on a decentralized discovery process that often doesn't rely on FDA-recognized evidence. Sometimes subsequent randomized controlled trials validate the off-label use, but often, the reverse happens. And off-label drug users risk adverse reactions.

To obtain evidence, patients, doctors, insurers, and even governments routinely rely on sources other than the FDA to certify the efficacy of off-label uses. Examples of non-FDA efficacy certification include drug compendia, *Consumer Reports*, foreign regulatory agencies, and medical journals. The federal government and all 56 state and territorial governments recognize multiple voluntary, private-sector efficacy certifications as reasonable alternatives to the FDA's seal of approval. Federal law requires the Medicare program to rely on specific privately compiled drug compendia to certify the efficacy of off-label uses. For instance, it directs Medicare to rely on "the American Hospital Formulary Service-Drug Information, the American Medical Association Drug Evaluations, the United States Pharmacopoeia Drug Information (or its successor publications), and other authoritative compendia as identified by the Secretary" for off-label indications of anticancer drugs.[9] Federal law further authorizes the Secretary of Health and Human Services (HHS) to designate additional compendia and medical journals on which Medicare must rely. The compendia named above have all gone out of print, so the secretary has designated alternative compendia as authoritative sources of efficacy certification of anticancer drugs.[10] Over time, HHS secretaries have accepted four compendia and more than a dozen medical journals as authorities on the efficacy of off-label uses. Federal law imposes similar requirements on state Medicaid programs.[11] Most state legislatures have enacted laws requiring private health insurers to cover off-label use of cancer drugs based on compendia listings.[12]

Even the FDA relied on a private third-party reviewer, the National Research Council of the National Academy of Sciences, to certify the efficacy of drugs between 1938 and 1962. And before 1938, the private sector carried out the responsibilities of the FDA. It remains uncertain how many additional private entities would presently handle these functions—and likely in a more efficient manner—if the FDA were not displacing them.

Drug Lag and Drug Loss

When Congress enacted the Kefauver-Harris Amendments, it created the twin problems of "drug lag" and "drug loss." Drug lag refers to the additional time that the FDA's proof-of-efficacy requirement forces consumers to wait before they may access a drug. Every day that the FDA adds to the drug development and approval process is a day that the agency denies consumers their right to self-medicate with that drug. Drug lag is cruelest to terminally ill patients, to whom it denies the right to try to save their lives by using drugs that have already been proven safe but are awaiting efficacy approval. Many seriously ill Americans die waiting for the FDA to approve drugs that regulators in other countries have already approved.[13]

Drug loss occurs when pharmaceutical manufacturers choose not to invest in finding new treatments that they do not believe can recoup the considerable cost of securing FDA approval. Drug loss denies consumers freedom to access drugs with a lower expected benefit-to-cost ratio than the FDA might accept or whose potential market is too small to recoup the cost of an FDA approval. The fact that drug loss denies manufacturers the freedom to bring those drugs to market makes it no less an infringement on consumers' right to self-medicate.

The high cost of the FDA's approval processes leads to higher drug prices. It also incentivizes manufacturers to market drugs as prescription-only so that they can charge higher prices to third-party payers covering prescription drugs to help recoup those costs.

The rising financial and delay costs of FDA regulation exacerbate both problems. Studies have found that the time required to take a drug through FDA-mandated clinical testing and marketing approval alone rose from 7.5 years (90.3 months) in the 1980s and 1990s to 8 years (96.3 months) in the 1990s and 2000s. These estimates do not count the preclinical phase of drug development, between the synthesis of a new chemical entity and human testing, which adds several years to the FDA approval process. And, presented in 2019 dollars, the average estimated cost of each new drug approval has risen from $523 million in 1987 to $1.2–1.8 billion in 2000 to $3.2 billion in 2013. The cost grew at an average annual real rate of 9.4 percent in the 1970s, 7.4 percent in the 1980s, and 8.5 percent from 1990 through the early 2010s.[14]

Rather than save lives, the Kefauver-Harris Amendments may cost lives. Keeping new drugs off the market until manufacturers conduct increasingly extensive clinical trials no doubt saves lives by preventing unsafe drugs from coming to market. Yet it also causes patients to suffer—and even die—while waiting for treatments to clear the FDA's approval process.

Dissatisfaction with the length of the FDA's approval process led to a national movement that spurred legislation at the state level and a federal "Right to Try" law in 2018. These laws allow some terminally ill patients to access drugs that the FDA is blocking from the market.[15] Patients such as five-year-old Jordan McLinn, whose diagnosis of Duchenne Muscular Dystrophy gives him a life expectancy of 20 years, or 30-year-old Amanda Wilcox, who has advanced-stage colon cancer, have sought to exercise their right to try potentially life-saving drugs that have not completed FDA-required clinical trials.[16] Regrettably, the government persists in encroaching upon the right of adults to self-medicate, relenting only when they are on the brink of death and facing a seemingly hopeless situation.

Medical Devices and the Right to Self-Test

The right to self-test is a corollary of the right to self-medicate and is integral to personal autonomy. A person must be able to acquire information about oneself and one's health status to give informed consent to treatment or to self-medicate.

During the COVID-19 pandemic's early days, the FDA's cumbersome regulatory process authorized a single government-monopoly coronavirus test, which was available in limited supply and produced by the Centers for Disease Control and Prevention (CDC). The FDA blocked patients from accessing private-sector and foreign-developed tests during the crucial weeks between when overseas public health authorities first identified the virus in December 2019 and when it started spreading throughout the United States in late January 2020. Meanwhile, when the Centers for Disease Control and Prevention rolled out the tests, they were defective, which forced the CDC to play catch-up and get new, corrected tests out to the public.[17]

In the meantime, other countries were already relying on tests developed by numerous private-sector companies and organizations operating under more liberal regulatory regimes. The World Health Organization distributed a test developed by a Berlin-based biotech firm to 57 countries, and China had five commercial tests on the market in January 2020. South Korea enacted a reform after suffering a devastating attack of Middle East Respiratory Syndrome (MERS) in 2015 that granted a nearly immediate approval of testing systems in the event of an emergency.[18]

While the rest of the world sought to enable and benefit from private-sector initiatives, the United States embraced a top-down command-and-control approach to the biomedical challenge, replete with red tape and poor communication with local public health officials. By March 2020, the FDA relaxed its stringent approval process and encouraged a rapid private-sector response. As an emergency measure, it relaxed its medical device approval process to allow state governments to approve COVID-19 tests for patients to use within their borders. As federal, state, and local health authorities rushed to get tests out to people who were suspected of having COVID-19 infection several weeks later than they could have, the infection spread and fatalities increased. Many people might have survived had the government not infringed on their right to self-test.[19]

In mid-November 2020, the FDA proudly announced that it had approved the first at-home self-administered test for COVID-19. Amidst the concern that asymptomatic carriers could unknowingly spread the virus, and with testing crucial to discriminate between those who could go to work and those who should quarantine, this announcement seemed like a beautiful breakthrough—until one read the fine print. It turned out that accessing the test, brand-named Lucira COVID-19 All-in-One Test Kit, required a prescription from a licensed health care practitioner. The FDA instructed clinicians only to prescribe the test to symptomatic patients. The agency did not want people to purchase and self-administer the test otherwise. This defeats the purpose of an at-home test and runs counter to the goal of restraining contagion, since presymptomatic patients can be contagious. One month later, the FDA approved an app-based at-home test called BinaxNOW. The FDA also required a prescription and for patients to have symptoms to access the test. The app-based telehealth provider reported findings to public health authorities.[20]

Around the same time, the FDA finally approved a different at-home test, Ellume, without a prescription requirement. However, the test used a mobile phone app to analyze a nasal swab and share the results with public health authorities who could then maintain surveillance. Self-administered at-home test kits were widely available from many manufacturers in Europe and Asia months before the FDA stopped blocking Americans from obtaining them.[21]

One can argue that, in a public health emergency, the government can require people to share their test results so that public health authorities can quarantine infected people. One can also argue for rationing tests that are in short supply during a public health emergency. However, one cannot justify denying people the right to obtain a test to learn about their health status.

The Food, Drug, and Cosmetic Act of 1938 gave the FDA the ability to regulate medical devices. The FDA defined medical devices as instruments or apparatuses used to diagnose, mitigate, treat, prevent, or cure a disease in humans and animals. But the FDCA only allowed the FDA to act against manufacturers for selling adulterated, misbranded, or unreliable devices after they had already been released into the market.

However, in 1972, the FDA stretched the meaning of "unreliable" when it recalled an at-home pregnancy test that was identical to the test used by physicians to diagnose pregnancy. The agency argued that women may not make decisions that are in the best interests of their health if they learn they are pregnant without a physician present. The manufacturer, Faraday, sued the agency. In 1974, the court ruled that the FDCA did not give the FDA the authority to regulate the test kit as a drug and that the FDA held the manufacturer to an impossible standard of "reliability."[22]

Congress broadened the scope of the FDA's regulatory authority over medical devices when it enacted the Medical Device Amendments to the FDCA in 1976. Among other things, the amendments required medical device manufacturers to gain premarket approval from the FDA, authorized the FDA to confirm that such devices were "safe" and "effective" and tasked the FDA with classifying them based on three levels of risk to which they subjected consumers. Class I devices are "low risk" and are "subject to general controls," such as product registration and monitoring. Class II devices are "moderate risk" and are subject to more controls to ensure safety and effectiveness. Class III devices are "high risk" and require more-detailed information, including clinical safety and efficacy studies, before the agency approves them.[23]

At-home tests pose little risk to the user. They usually involve using a swabbing device to sample the nasal or oral cavities or to obtain a body fluid sample. It is more of an issue for the FDA whether at-home tests are accurate or efficacious. And in recent years FDA regulators have stretched the meaning of efficacy to include how a patient uses the knowledge obtained from a test. However, how a person uses information is a normative matter—a value judgment—that should be left to the individual, not the government, to decide.

HIV Tests

During the HIV/AIDS crisis in the 1980s, the FDA resisted manufacturers' efforts to develop at-home HIV tests. While it accepted pre-market approval applications in 1986 and 1987, it ended the practice in 1988, making it clear that the agency was only interested in evaluating blood collection kits that manufacturers designed "for professional use only" and for use "within a health care environment," such as a hospital, medical clinic, or physician's office. The agency indicated publicly that it was concerned about how consumers would understand and react to positive at-home test results. The agency feared, for instance, that some patients might consider suicide rather than treatment. It believed the risk of such a reaction would be lower if a professional delivered the information in a health care setting. After numerous AIDS advocacy groups pleaded with the agency, the FDA lifted its ban on at-home collection kit applications in 1995, but it didn't lift its ban on at-home self-administered test kit applications until 2005. The agency finally approved the first at-home self-administered HIV test kit in 2012.[24] It is impossible to estimate the number of people who unknowingly transmitted HIV because the government did not permit them to self-test with at-home kits.

For the same reasons, the FDA has been slow to allow screening for specific diseases using direct-to-consumer genetic test kits such as 23andMe.[25] It is an affront to patient autonomy to deny adults the right to seek information about their health by getting tested. It adds insult to injury by infringing on this right for paternalistic reasons.

Meanwhile, most states allow their residents to patronize freestanding clinical laboratories, such as those run by Quest and Labcorp, and purchase direct-to-consumer tests without a prescription or requisition from a government-licensed health care clinician. Some health insurance plans will only reimburse the cost of lab tests if a clinician prescribes them. However, according to a Johns Hopkins University "Survey of Direct-to-Consumer Statutes and Regulations," 25 states plus the District of Columbia have no barriers to consumers exercising their right to test, 12 states restrict the right to test for some but not all conditions, and 13 states completely block patients from direct-to-consumer clinical laboratory testing.[26] Thus, some state governments respect adults' right to test and use test information more than the federal government does.

The Journey to Self-Governance

Ideally, Congress should end the FDA's power to deny consumers their right to self-test and self-medicate through its power over the drug and medical device approval process. That power stems from the Food, Drug, and Cosmetic Act and its amendments, which require all new drugs, all generic drugs, all forms of manufacturer speech about new uses for existing drugs, and all medical devices to receive the FDA's approval before going to market. So long as Congress allows the FDA to act as a paternalistic gatekeeper between consumers and drugs, the agency will err on the side of delaying and denying consumers access to new products and new information.[27] The FDA has an incentive to be overly cautious because any unsafe drugs that reach patients could lead to public criticism of the agency. However, the public cannot know of the potential benefits that are lost when a drug or device doesn't come to market, as they can't see the individuals who would have benefited from them, so the FDA faces little to no criticism for not approving or delaying certain drugs.

Private-sector organizations can perform the same function as the FDA in certifying that drugs and devices are safe and effective. The crucial difference is that private certification organizations can provide consumers with the information they need to make educated treatment decisions but cannot deny them access to medical care.

Absent the FDA monopoly on initial safety and efficacy certification, we would likely witness a proliferation of efficient alternative standards. Alongside existing informal certification mechanisms, medical societies—including specialty societies—might reenter the market and take charge of safety and efficacy certifications for drugs and devices within their fields.

Health plans are driven by strong incentives and would actively support certification bodies, or even perform that role themselves. Their coverage decisions could inform enrollees about the efficacy and cost-effectiveness of various drugs and devices. Integrated prepaid group plans, such as Kaiser Permanente, would hold a significant advantage, with their prepayment model encouraging them to fund research to distinguish between effective and ineffective drugs and devices. Additionally, their fully integrated delivery systems would enable them to conduct safety and efficacy studies.

In a competitive market where the federal government respects the right to self-medicate and self-test, the persistent issues of drug lag and drug loss would dissipate. Unnecessary regulations would no longer hinder consumers' access to drugs and devices. Individuals would be free to choose drugs and devices based on their benefit versus cost assessments after considering the quality of evidence regarding efficacy and cost-effectiveness.

As with a government-mandated prescription from a physician, an FDA approval can lead consumers to make less careful drug-consumption decisions than they would in its absence. A competitive market for drug certification, where different certifiers reach different conclusions about the same drug, would educate consumers that all drugs carry risks and that safety and efficacy are not binary concepts, but can be mutually reinforcing. A competitive market for safety and efficacy certification would allow private certifiers to develop and use multiple graduated categories that are better at educating consumers and clinicians about the benefits and costs of drugs, the strengths and weaknesses of the evidence for those benefits and costs, and the nature of drugs, health, and risk.

As an intermediate step, Congress could pass legislation giving automatic approval to drugs and medical devices available in other developed countries.[28] Under reciprocal approval, the government allows consumers to access drugs and devices that designated foreign government certification bodies have approved. ("Reciprocal approval" is an inapt term since the foreign certification entities do not need to certify FDA-approved products in return.) Reciprocal approval of all drugs and all devices bearing a CE marking (from the French term *conformité européenne*, translated as "European conformity"), which designates that a device meets European Union standards, already exists between the European Union member states, Iceland, Liechtenstein, and Norway.[29]

In November 2022, the Swiss parliament enacted legislation allowing Swiss residents to access FDA-approved devices.[30] Previously the Swiss government only allowed its residents to use CE-labeled devices. Australia began permitting patients and doctors to access FDA-approved medical devices in 2018 and has allowed them to use EU-approved devices for several years.[31] Israel permits its residents to use drugs and devices that the governments of the United States, the European Union, Australia, and Canada have approved.[32]

According to one study, recognizing drug approvals by regulatory bodies in Canada and Europe between 2000 and 2010 would have given US consumers quicker access to 37 "novel" drugs for which "no other FDA-approved prescription medicine had the same mechanism of action," including 10 drugs treating mostly orphan diseases (those that receive little or no research funding) "for which no alternative therapy was available in the USA." Such recognition would have allowed American consumers to access those drugs a median of 13.6 months earlier.[33]

States should not place legal obstacles in the way of patients exercising their right to self-test. All states should remove any remaining requirements that patients get permission from state-licensed health care practitioners to access clinical laboratories for health status information.

Knowing that some individuals would inevitably self-medicate in ways that harm their health should not delay reform. Americans routinely exercise their right to refuse potentially beneficial medical treatments.

The utilitarian argument for eliminating the government monopoly on drug and device approval is not that manufacturers and consumers of pharmaceuticals will never make harmful mistakes. The government is now making far more harmful mistakes than a free consumer populace aided by price competition, quality competition, third-party certification, innovation, greater health literacy, and the threat of tort liability would make.[34]

The onus is not on those advocating to restore individuals' right to make their own health care decisions. It lies with those who would preserve laws upholding government violations of personal autonomy. The individual-rights argument for eliminating the FDA's monopoly is that the government has no moral authority to interfere in those decisions in the first place.

CHAPTER 6

The War on (Some) Drugs

Since the beginning of the 20th century, the government has viewed people as being immoral if they choose to consume certain psychoactive substances, such as alcohol, cocaine, opiates, opioids, and psychedelic drugs. Policymakers have given short shrift to the individual's fundamental right to self-medicate. A right that America's Founding generation revered as sacrosanct has been ignored by policymakers who are intent to impose their idea of moral and healthful drug consumption on the adult population.

In 1920, the federal government imposed a nationwide ban on the production and sale of ethyl alcohol (ethanol) for human consumption, except for medicinal or religious purposes. Alcohol prohibition created a wave of crime and corruption as illegal alcohol dealers, commonly called "bootleggers," engaged in violent battles over distribution territories and bribed politicians and police to overlook their activities. Bootleggers often fortified alcohol with methanol to increase its potency, which often caused blindness and death. The government ordered that stocks of ethanol that were legally allowed for commercial use be denatured with benzene and other poisons to discourage the recreational use of them. Federally ordered denatured alcohol was responsible for thousands of deaths during the Prohibition

Era. Seymour Lowman, the assistant secretary of the Treasury who was in charge of enforcing alcohol prohibition, famously said that if people were "dying off fast from poison 'hooch'" it might frighten the rest of the public to stay sober.[1] By 1933, the public soured on alcohol prohibition. Congress repealed the federal ban, leaving it to the individual states to decide on the matter. In 1966, Mississippi became the last state to repeal statewide prohibition.[2]

As alcohol prohibition faded from memory, society came to view recreational alcohol consumption as acceptable behavior and approached alcohol addiction as a health problem deserving empathy and compassion. Unfortunately, government policymakers failed to absorb two of the biggest lessons of alcohol prohibition. One of the biggest lessons is that when the government tries to prohibit adults from consuming a substance, whether for enjoyment or to self-medicate, people will find ways to obtain it and purveyors will find ways to sell it to them. Another big lesson is that prohibition creates a deadly but thriving underground market. Government prohibition drives the supply and demand underground, where consumers cannot be sure about the potency, quality, and purity of the substances they buy, and competing marketers can only resolve their disputes through violence.

Federal and state governments began to develop an expanding system of drug prohibition in 1914, when Congress passed the Harrison Narcotics Act. Following its passage, the government started by banning drugs such as opium, opium derivatives, and cocaine. It has continued adding a growing number of psychoactive substances to the list and incarcerates people for buying, selling, possessing, or consuming these products.[3]

As with alcohol, many prohibitionists exploited racist and xenophobic sentiments among the broader population. Progressives concerned about alcohol's unhealthful effects aligned with racist and xenophobic organizations such as the Ku Klux Klan, which sought to control Catholics, immigrants, and African Americans, whom they associated with alcohol use, by promoting alcohol prohibition.[4] Opium prohibitionists tapped into anti-Chinese xenophobia.[5] Myths about "cocaine-crazed negroes," who were impervious to bullets and who were able to take long and difficult jobs away from white laborers, fueled public support of cocaine prohibition.[6] Eric Schlosser writes that advocates of cannabis prohibition began referring to it as marijuana, a term used by Mexican migrants, which they claimed gave users "superhuman strength" and a "lust for blood." They warned that this dangerous drug was popular among "African-Americans, jazz musicians, prostitutes, and underworld whites."[7]

Those in power have continued to use prohibition as a means of controlling marginalized and disfavored groups into modern times. Former assistant to President Richard Nixon for domestic affairs John Ehrlichman famously confessed to journalist Dan Baum in a 1994 interview for *Harper's*:

> You want to know what this was really all about? . . . The Nixon campaign in 1968, and the Nixon White House after that, had two enemies: the antiwar left and black people. You understand what I'm saying? We knew we couldn't make it illegal to be either against the war or black, but by getting the public to associate the hippies with marijuana and blacks with heroin, and then criminalizing both heavily, we could disrupt those communities. We could arrest their leaders, raid their homes, break up their meetings, and vilify them night after night on the evening news. Did we know we were lying about the drugs? Of course we did.[8]

This "war on drugs," as Nixon named it in 1971, has destructively intruded on the patient-doctor relationship.[9] Government and law enforcement increasingly surveil and influence the way doctors treat pain, psychoactive substance use, and substance use disorder. Drug prohibition has happened in two discernible waves: Drug War I and Drug War II.

Drug War I occurred after Congress enacted the Harrison Narcotics Act in 1914, which permitted doctors to prescribe opioids to treat their patients. A wave of arrests and prosecutions of thousands of doctors ensued as agents of the US Treasury Department, empowered to enforce the act, took it upon themselves to define legitimate medical practice.

Drug War II began in the 1970s with government-funded education/indoctrination campaigns that caused both doctors and patients to fear opioids for their addictive and overdose potential. Later, as the scientific literature led medical specialty organizations and government health officials to overcome this apprehension and take the treatment of pain more seriously, opioid prescribing increased considerably.

By 2006, federal regulatory agencies perceived what they called an "opioid crisis" and mistakenly attributed it to doctors overprescribing opioids and generating a growing population of opioid addicts. This formed the basis for an even more massive intrusion of federal and state power into the privacy of medical records, patient-doctor confidentiality, and how doctors are allowed to use scientific and professional knowledge to practice medicine. Medical decisionmaking came increasingly under the purview of law enforcement, sparking a new wave of arrests and prosecutions. Despite government and law enforcement efforts, the overdose death rate from using illicit substances continues to climb, and the drugs responsible grow ever more potent.[10]

Opiates and Opioids

Many policymakers and opinion leaders use the words "opioids" and "opiates" interchangeably, but the two words have different meanings.

Opiates refers to drugs that manufacturers derive directly from the opium plant, *Papaver somniferum*. Opiates are natural drugs. These drugs include opium, morphine, and codeine. *Opioids* are opiates that chemists have modified, changing their pharmacologic properties so they affect patients differently. By adding molecules to existing opiates, chemists create *semi-synthetic opioids*. Semi-synthetic opioids include oxycodone, hydrocodone, hydromorphone (Dilaudid), and diamorphine (heroin). However, chemists can also manufacture drugs with opioid properties without using natural opiates. Such *synthetic opioids* include fentanyl, methadone, tramadol, and nitazenes. When the CDC reports on opioid-related overdose deaths, it categorizes them as "natural and semi-synthetic," "methadone," "synthetic opioids excluding methadone," and "heroin."[11]

The Overdose Crisis Didn't Begin in the Early 21st Century

Researchers at the University of Pittsburgh School of Public Health used data from the CDC to determine that the overdose death rate has been rising exponentially since at least the late 1970s, with different drugs dominating as the leading cause of overdose deaths at different times (see figure 6.1).[12] A 2019 report by the US Congressional Joint Economic Committee traced the beginning of the rise in overdose deaths to as far back as 1959.[13] A 2022 study reported in the *Journal of the American Medical Association* suggests that the country may be heading toward an even more significant wave of overdose deaths from new drug combinations.[14] However, in May 2024 the Centers for Disease Control and Prevention reported a 3 percent drop in US overdose deaths in 2023, the first annual decrease since 2018.[15]

The surge in overdose deaths that caught the attention of policymakers and public health authorities in the early 21st century has continued despite government policies that focused on reducing the rate of opioids that doctors prescribe to treat patients in pain. Those policies led to a 60 percent drop in opioid prescribing from 2011 to 2020.[16] Additionally, the Drug Enforcement Administration (DEA)

FIGURE 6.1

Mortality rates from unintentional drug overdoses for individual drugs and all drugs

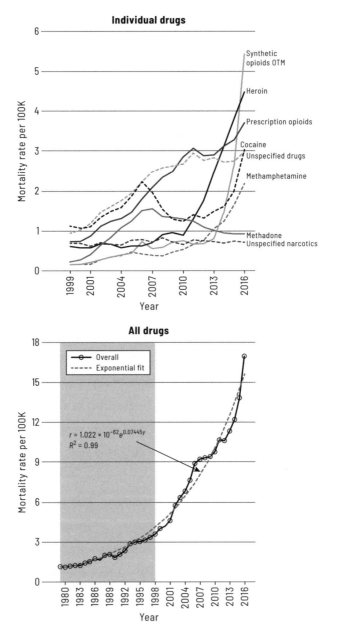

Source: Hawre Jalal et al., "Changing Dynamics of the Drug Overdose Epidemic in the United States from 1979 through 2016," *Science* 361, no. 6408 (September 21, 2018): eaau1184.
Note: Detailed data from individual drugs are only available from 1999 to 2016, while additional data are available since 1979 for all drugs (this area is greyed out). The exponential equation and fit are shown for all drugs.
r = overall mortality rate; y = year; OTM = synthetic opioids other than methadone. This category includes fentanyl and its analogues.

placed quotas on the manufacturing of all types of prescription opioids, ratcheting those quotas downward year after year. By 2019 the
reduction in the prescribing rate led the DEA to announce that less
than 1 percent of controlled substances distributed to retail purchas-
ers were finding their way into the underground market.[17]

Prohibitionists believed that doctors caused the 21st-century
overdose crisis by inadvertently addicting their patients to opioids,
creating a population of zombie-like drug seekers who fell victim to
dangerous black-market drugs. However, data from the National Survey on Drug Use and Health (conducted each year since 2002 by the
Substance Abuse and Mental Health Services Administration) and
the CDC show no significant change in the percentage of persons aged
12 and above who engaged in "past month nonmedical use of prescription pain relievers" or who developed "pain reliever use disorder in the
past year" from 2002 to 2014—a period when the prescription volume
almost doubled.[18] Furthermore, the National Survey on Drug Use and
Health finds that the per capita addiction rate among adults has been
essentially stable (see figure 6.2).

In the early part of the 21st century, people using drugs nonmedi-
cally or to self-medicate for physical or psychic pain chose prescription
pain pills obtained in the black market. Many state and county prosecutors believed that the semi-synthetic opioid OxyContin (slow-release
oxycodone) was a main driver of overdoses among nonmedical opioid
users. However, researchers reported in the *Yale Law and Policy Review*
in 2023 that "only 9.0 percent of all nonmedical opioid users in 2001
reported ever using OxyContin during their lifetime."[19]

As governments at all levels pressured health care practitioners to
reduce opioid prescribing and DEA quotas on opioid production took
effect, the supply of black-market prescription pain pills decreased.
Users turned to heroin (diamorphine), which was cheap and abundant.
Heroin-related overdose deaths climbed as deaths from prescription

FIGURE 6.2

Trends in substance use disorder in the past year among adults aged 18 or older, by selected types of substances, 2002–2014

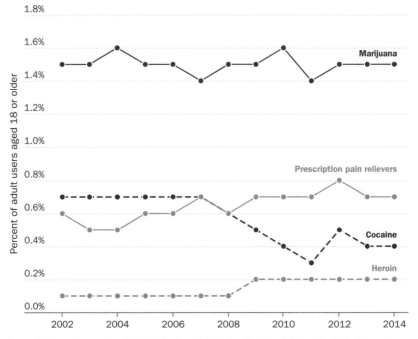

Source: Substance Abuse and Mental Health Services Administration, Center for Behavioral Health Statistics and Quality, National Surveys on Drug Use and Health, 2002 to 2005, 2006 to 2010 (revised March 2012), and 2011 to 2014.

pain pill overdoses receded. In 2012, heroin purveyors began adding in the synthetic opioid fentanyl, a legal prescription drug they illicitly produced in underground labs. Fentanyl-related overdose deaths started rising in 2012. As show in figure 6.3, they eclipsed deaths from heroin and black-market prescription pain pills in 2016. By 2017, fentanyl was associated with more than 50 percent of opioid-related overdose deaths. By 2022, it was involved in roughly 90 percent.[20]

Most opioid-related overdose deaths associated with nonmedical use involve multiple other drugs, including alcohol, benzodiazepines, cocaine, and methamphetamine. In New York City, 97 percent of opioid-related overdose deaths in 2016 involved more than one drug, including illicit drugs such as cocaine and methamphetamine.[21]

FIGURE 6.3

Fentanyl has dwarfed prescription opioids as the dominant cause of opioid-related overdose deaths

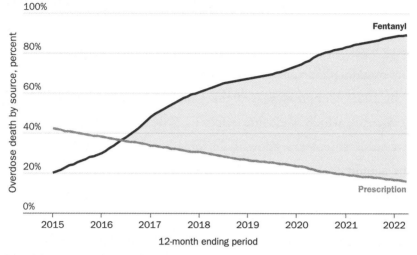

Source: F. B. Ahmad et al., "Provisional Drug Overdose Death Counts," National Vital Statistics System, Center for Disease Control and Prevention, October 12, 2022.
Note: The sum of the percentage of fentanyl and prescription opioids can equal more than 100 percent because an overdose death may include a combination of the two.

In 2017, 86 percent of opioid-related overdose deaths in New York City involved heroin or fentanyl, 49 percent involved cocaine, and just 14 percent involved prescription opioids.[22] National data from the CDC reveal that 68 percent of overdose deaths involving prescription opioids in 2017 involved multiple other drugs as well.[23]

Methamphetamine, Cocaine, Cannabis, and Other Prohibited Drugs

Methamphetamine

Like fentanyl, methamphetamine (meth) is a legal prescription drug that drug dealers can easily synthesize in a basement lab. Sold under the brand name Desoxyn, methamphetamine was one of the early drugs that doctors prescribed to treat attention-deficit/hyperactivity disorder and is also prescribed for narcolepsy.[24] People have been using methamphetamine for decades to improve their focus and attention, to keep them awake, or for recreation, even though the government will not allow them to.

A thriving black market in meth led to an epidemic of meth-related deaths and prohibition-related violent crime.[25] Meth "cooks" were using legal over-the-counter drugs containing the effective decongestant pseudoephedrine to manufacture meth in their labs.

In 2005, Congress passed the Combat Methamphetamine Epidemic Act, which went into effect in 2006. In addition to funding law enforcement crackdowns on local homegrown meth labs, the law sought to prevent the diversion of pseudoephedrine into the black-market meth labs. The law authorized the DEA to order all oral pseudoephedrine medications to be sold behind the counter. The law required pharmacists to record the personal identification of patients who purchase a pseudoephedrine product.[26] The DEA then placed strict limits on the dose and number of pseudoephedrine-containing products patients were allowed to obtain within a 30-day time frame. Oregon and Mississippi lawmakers went even further. Those states required patients to get a doctor's prescription to purchase oral pseudoephedrine. Both states have since repealed their prescription requirements.[27]

The new law required Sudafed, a popular and effective brand of pseudoephedrine decongestant, and other drugs to be placed behind the counter. However, people can purchase Sudafed PE and other nasal decongestions over the counter without restrictions.[28] Sudafed PE substitutes phenylephrine for pseudoephedrine (thus the "PE"). Most other makers of pseudoephedrine-containing cold and allergy remedies substituted phenylephrine as well to enable consumers to avoid the inconvenience, scrutiny, and even the stigma attached to buying pseudoephedrine from behind the counter.[29]

In September 2023, an FDA advisory panel reported that oral phenylephrine does not reduce nasal congestion. (The FDA certified phenylephrine as safe and effective in the 1970s.) Unlike pseudo-ephedrine, digestive enzymes break down the drug when it is taken orally, and it doesn't work any better than a placebo.[30] Meanwhile, while millions of nasal congestion sufferers wasted their money on phenylephrine products, the Mexican drug cartels filled the void in the black market that DEA raids on local meth labs had created and quickly realized that they could make a more potent form of meth more efficiently using the industrial chemical phenyl-2-propanone (P2P).[31] While people still must show identification and register for DEA surveillance when they buy a pseudoephedrine product behind the counter, meth-related deaths per 100,000 people have increased by 1,400 percent between 2006 (when the Combat Methamphetamine Epidemic Act went into effect) and 2020.[32]

In a tragic irony, the FDA and the DEA combined to make millions of people with colds, allergies, and other causes of severe congestion waste their money on de facto placebos and go without relief for decades, while driving Mexican drug cartels to discover more-effective ways to make more-potent forms of meth, causing meth-related deaths to skyrocket.

Cocaine

To eradicate the thriving underground cocaine market that was based in Colombia, the US government implemented Plan Colombia in 2000. This involved the US and Colombian militaries collaborating to root out the Colombian drug cartels and Colombian narco-terrorists and addressing the social problems they caused.[33] As a result, Central America became the next node of drug trafficking and crime. Then it moved north to Mexico. Later, after the capture of "El Chapo" Guzman, the leader of Mexico's dominant Sinaloa drug cartel, a multiyear surge of violence followed as new contenders battled to control the lucrative drug routes into America.[34] Like water in a boulder-laden creek, prohibited drugs keep finding their way downstream to consumers despite the federal government's determined efforts. Today, cocaine remains cheap and abundant, and increasing numbers of people are consuming it.[35] More than 28,000 people died of cocaine-related overdoses by mid-2023, a record high.[36]

Cannabis

People have been using cannabis medicinally for millennia. The historical record of medicinal cannabis dates as far back as 2800 BCE.[37] Sir William Osler, considered by many medical educators to be the father of modern medicine, wrote numerous articles and an entry in his 1916 textbook *Principles and Practice of Medicine*, proclaiming cannabis as the drug of choice to treat migraines.[38] Yet today, as a result of the Controlled Substances Act of 1970, the DEA classifies cannabis as a Schedule I drug that has "no currently accepted medical use and a high potential for abuse."[39]

In the 1930s, Harry Anslinger, then head of the Federal Bureau of Narcotics, began waging war on cannabis as it became obvious that the American public was losing its stomach for alcohol prohibition. He employed racist tropes to fuel his campaign, repeatedly referring to cannabis as marijuana to invoke the drug's popularity among Mexican immigrants. He also claimed that "marijuana causes white women to seek sexual relations with Negroes, entertainers and any others," and that "reefer makes darkies think they're as good as white men."[40] His efforts led Congress to pass the Marijuana Tax Act of 1937, the first federal move toward cannabis prohibition.[41] Congress repealed the act in 1969 and included cannabis prohibition in the more comprehensive Controlled Substances Act of 1970.[42]

Federal and state law enforcement continue putting people in cages for possessing, using, or selling cannabis. According to research published by the American Civil Liberties Union, state-level law enforcement arrested more than six million people for cannabis possession between 2010 and 2018, with African Americans disproportionately arrested despite there being equal percentages of black people and white people who consume cannabis.[43] A felony conviction for choosing to grow, sell, or ingest a plant can ruin a person's future. Many employers will not hire people with felony records, and many state occupational and professional licensing boards will deny felony convicts an opportunity to earn an honest living.[44]

It is much less harmful to consume cannabis than it is to consume alcohol.[45] There is no lethal dose of cannabis, and no history of anyone dying from consuming too much of it.[46] Cannabis is also less likely to lead to violent behavior than alcohol.[47] The main active ingredient in cannabis, tetrahydrocannabinol (THC) does not cause respiratory depression.[48]

In 2022, 132 million people in the United States reported that they defied the government by consuming cannabis at least once in their lifetime.[49] A Gallup survey in late 2023 found that 70 percent of adults favored the repeal of cannabis prohibition.[50]

Beginning in the 1990s, citizens began passing ballot initiatives legalizing cannabis for medicinal use in certain states, and legislators in other states began legalizing medicinal cannabis as well. Beginning in the early 21st century, state governments began permitting people to consume cannabis for recreational use. By the end of 2023, governments in 38 states, three US territories, and the District of Columbia enabled people to self-medicate with cannabis.[51] At the end of 2023, 24 states, two US territories, and the District of Columbia removed obstacles to people consuming cannabis for pleasure.[52]

Yet federal cannabis prohibition remains in place, creating legal obstacles to financial transactions and interstate commerce between legal cannabis retailers and consumers. Although President Joseph Biden pardoned the roughly 6,500 people with federal felony convictions for simple cannabis possession in October 2022, he continued to oppose repealing cannabis prohibition but signaled he was amenable to the idea of rescheduling cannabis as a controlled prescription medication, meaning that people would not be able to obtain it without a prescription.[53]

The *New York Times* reported in early 2024 that scientists at the FDA and the National Institute on Drug Abuse (NIDA) recommended that the DEA reschedule cannabis as a Schedule III drug.[54] The DEA defines Schedule III drugs as having a potential for abuse that is less than drugs in either Schedule I or II and whose abuse may lead to moderate or low physical dependence or high psychological dependence.[55] The *Times* article stated that FDA and NIDA scientists told the DEA that "the likelihood of serious outcomes is low" from chronic cannabis consumption and that "'there is some scientific support' for therapeutic uses of marijuana, including treatment for anorexia, pain, and nausea and vomiting related to chemotherapy."[56] The scientific review led the FDA to recommend to the DEA that it reschedule cannabis to Schedule III. On April 30, 2024, the DEA announced that it intends to reschedule cannabis.[57]

However, until the FDA approves cannabis for medical use, rescheduling will have little impact except to make it easier to conduct clinical research and allow retailers in states where it is legal to access financial services and take advantage of certain business tax deductions. Even if the FDA approves cannabis for medicinal use, federal law will still ban adults from obtaining or consuming cannabis without first getting a prescription.[58]

Psychedelics

Psychedelics were another category of drugs with great therapeutic potential that fell into disfavor by government authorities because it was popular with members of the 1960s counterculture, many of whom protested America's involvement in the war in Vietnam and advocated for civil rights and sexual liberation. Psychedelic drugs encompass a wide range of natural and synthetic drugs. Natural psychedelics include mushrooms containing psilocybin, mescaline from peyote cactus, dimethyltryptamine (DMT) from ayahuasca vines, and ibogaine from the iboga shrub. Synthetic psychedelics include lysergic acid diethylamide (LSD), or "acid," and 3,4-methylenedioxymethamphetamine (MDMA), or "ecstasy" and "Molly." People who consume psychedelics frequently can develop tolerance, but psychedelics are not addictive.[59]

Clinicians, primarily anesthesiologists and certified registered nurse anesthetists, have been using ketamine, another type of psychedelic, for several decades as an anesthetic agent. The DEA classifies the drug as Schedule III. The drug creates a dissociative state by disconnecting patients' mental processes from their pain perception. The drug is particularly useful in anesthesia for pediatric patients and third-degree burn victims. In recent years, mental health therapists and other clinicians have begun conducting sessions with patients using ketamine to treat depression and other mental disorders. People can take the drug orally, intravenously, or by intramuscular injection. However, because the FDA has not approved clinicians' use of the drug for these purposes, they are using the drug off-label.[60] In 2019, the FDA approved a ketamine derivative, esketamine (brand name Spravato), as a prescription nasal spray to treat depression. The FDA will only allow patients to take the drug with a certified physician or nurse practitioner supervising them in the practitioner's office or at a clinic.[61] The agency will not allow patients to self-administer the drug at home and check in with the doctor's office. In recent years, people have been obtaining ketamine on the black market and using the drug recreationally as a party drug or to self-medicate.[62]

Many states began prohibiting psychedelics in the 1960s, and after Congress passed the Controlled Substances Act in 1970, the DEA placed most psychedelic drugs on Schedule I. Before the DEA added psychedelics to Schedule I, researchers had conducted thousands of clinical studies that suggested the psychedelics had great potential for treating a range of mental health disorders.[63] The DEA added MDMA to Schedule I in 1985, after the drug became popular among rave concertgoers who called the drug "ecstasy."[64]

By placing psychedelics on Schedule I, the DEA made it very difficult for researchers to get permission from the government to conduct clinical studies. Nevertheless, recent research shows that psychotherapy with psychedelics, including psilocybin, MDMA, and LSD, appears to be effective in treating post-traumatic stress disorder (PTSD), tobacco and alcohol addiction, and clinical depression. In June 2023, the FDA published guidance on clinical trials with psychedelic drugs, including psilocybin, LSD, and MDMA. Unfortunately, in June 2024, an FDA advisory panel recommended against approving MDMA to treat PTSD by a vote of 9–2, and the FDA followed the panel's advice in August 2024.[65] As with cannabis, several states and municipalities are defying federal prohibition by legalizing both natural and synthetic psychedelics.[66]

When the DEA placed psychedelics on Schedule I, it squelched decades of promising clinical research. More than 50 years later, the government might, someday soon, let people get prescriptions to seek relief from the misery of PTSD (which has likely increased in prevalence since the wars in Iraq and Afghanistan), clinical depression, and substance use disorder.[67] Imagine how many people would have benefited during the past half-century had the government respected their autonomy and their right to self-medicate.

The "Iron Law of Prohibition"

In 1986, Richard Cowan applied what economists call the Alchian-Allen Effect to the prohibition of alcohol, cannabis, and other illicit substances. Cowan noted that as law enforcement on a substance became more intense, the potency of the prohibited substances increased; he called this principle the "iron law of prohibition."[68] Drug prohibition incentivizes the creation of more-potent forms of the drug to create better efficiencies for the business model because smaller packages of the drug make smuggling easier. Drug dealers can subdivide potent forms into several portions to sell, improving the dealers' risk/benefit ratio. The iron law explains why bootleggers smuggled whiskey instead of beer or wine during alcohol prohibition, why cannabis has increased in tetrahydrocannabinol concentration, and why powdered cocaine brought on crack cocaine. It's also why cracking down on black-market prescription pain pills brought on heroin and why cracking down on heroin brought on fentanyl.

The iron law of prohibition explains why the veterinary tranquilizer xylazine (users call it "tranq") is emerging as a new threat. Drug dealers are adding xylazine to the illicit fentanyl that they smuggle into the country and sell on the black market.[69] They also mix it with other illegal drugs, such as cocaine and methamphetamine. The sedative properties of the drug greatly enhance the narcotic effects of opioids.

Xylazine is a muscle relaxant and sedative often used in veterinary anesthesia. It has strong alpha-adrenergic properties, which cause constriction of the blood vessels, thus dramatically reducing the blood supply to the soft tissues near the injection site and often causing the tissue to die and creating infected ulcerations on the users' limbs. Sometimes the infections are severe enough to require life-saving limb amputations. While xylazine users can develop a physical dependency, the drug is more dangerous because the opioid overdose antidote naloxone does not reverse the respiratory depression seen with xylazine overdoses.[70]

Toxicology studies found xylazine mixed with illicit drugs starting in the early 2000s. In 2012, researchers at the University of Puerto Rico reported it mixed in with cocaine and heroin.[71] In recent years xylazine has infiltrated the United States and Canada.[72] The DEA reports that it found xylazine in 23 percent of fentanyl powder and 7 percent of fentanyl pills that the agency seized in 2022.[73]

And the problem hasn't stopped with "tranq." In 2019, health departments in Europe and the United States began seeing the synthetic opioid nitazene in overdose toxicology studies. In September 2022, the Tennessee Department of Health reported that nitazene-related overdose deaths increased fourfold between 2019 and 2021.[74] Nitazenes are derived from benzimidazole, a compound used in anti-fungal agents, antacids such as omeprazole and pantoprazole, and for drugs used to treat roundworms and flatworms in humans.

The Swiss drugmaker CIBA developed nitazenes in the 1950s but never brought them to market. Some nitazenes may be 20 times more potent than fentanyl. Fortunately, naloxone reverses nitazene overdoses, although it might require multiple doses. Most health departments haven't been testing for nitazenes, so we remain unaware if nitazenes are becoming more prevalent among black-market drugs. However, the UK press reported in late 2023 that nitazenes were showing up in toxicology studies in all parts of Britain. Often nitazenes contaminate black-market benzodiazepines, such as Xanax. London police seized 150,000 nitazene tablets in October 2023, the biggest haul of nitazenes to date.[75] Like fentanyl and its analogs, nitazene and its derivatives are relatively easy to synthesize in underground labs. Unlike fentanyl, nitazenes have never undergone clinical trials and doctors have never used them to treat patients. Therefore, medical experts know very little about the strength, drug interactions, and side effects of nitazene and its derivatives. This makes the drug's appearance in the black market potentially catastrophic.

Addiction and Dependence Are Not the Same Thing and That's Important

Misinformation regarding the difference between addiction and dependence animates many drug prohibitionists. People often conflate the two or use the two terms interchangeably, but they represent distinctly different phenomena. Dependency refers to the physiological adaptation to the drug to such an extent that abrupt cessation can cause a physical withdrawal reaction. Addiction is a behavioral disorder characterized by compulsive use despite negative consequences. People who are addicted to a substance still feel compelled to use the substance even when they are no longer physically dependent.[76] However, addiction is a behavioral disorder that can also apply to activities. For example, the American Psychiatric Association's (APA) *Diagnostic and Statistical Manual of Mental Disorders* lists gambling disorder as an addictive disorder.[77] The APA requires further peer-reviewed research before it adds other repetitive behavioral problems to the list of behavioral addictions that it currently lists among "impulse control disorders," such as hypersexuality (sex addiction), shopping addiction, and kleptomania.[78]

Many classes of drugs can cause physical dependency and withdrawal reactions when people suddenly stop using them after a prolonged period. Examples include beta-blockers (used to treat high blood pressure), anti-epileptic drugs, and antidepressants. Opioids cause dependence as well. Opioid withdrawal is rarely fatal, although it can be.[79] Withdrawal from some drugs, such as beta-blockers, can more often be fatal.[80] Some psychoactive drugs, such as cocaine or methamphetamine, generate only minor *physical* dependence and withdrawal symptoms, though they cause significant *psychological* dependence and withdrawal.[81]

People who are addicted to a substance are usually also physiologically dependent. However, people who have developed physiological dependence on a substance are not necessarily addicted. It is preposterous to refer to a person who is physiologically dependent on a beta-blocker as a "beta-blocker addict." Yet it is common to hear even medical professionals refer to people who develop a physiological dependency on a government-controlled substance—for example, hospitalized patients maintained on morphine for several weeks—as being addicted to the drug. Stigma is attached to government-controlled psychoactive substances, which stems from lawmakers' moralizing when they decide to let the government control those substances.

People with addiction or substance use disorder almost always have a history of childhood trauma, and a majority also have psycho-neurological comorbidities.[82] These comorbidities may include one or more of the following: attention-deficit/hyperactivity disorder, depression, bipolar disorder, generalized anxiety disorder, PTSD, and obsessive-compulsive disorder.[83] Genetic vulnerabilities play a role in 40 to 60 percent of people who develop addiction.[84] Addiction also involves epigenetic mechanisms.[85] Yet, as Nora Volkow and Thomas McLellan, the director of the National Institute on Drug Abuse and the founder of the Treatment Research Institute, respectively, wrote in 2016, "Unlike tolerance and physical dependence, addiction is not a predictable result of opioid prescribing. Addiction occurs in only a small percentage of persons who are exposed to opioids—even among those with preexisting vulnerabilities."[86]

It is paternalistic for the government to prohibit people from selling, buying, or consuming drugs—even if the prohibition is limited to certain kinds of drugs. It assaults individuals' autonomy and their right to self-medicate.

Moreover, governments cannot stop people from using drugs. Governments can only make drug use more dangerous by driving it underground into an unregulated, and sometimes deadly, black market. Many of the drugs discussed in this chapter would be less harmful to health than legal ones, such as alcohol and tobacco, if people could obtain them in a legal market. The government has blood on its hands. The blood is not only from drug overdose victims, but also from victims of violent crimes, because prohibition attracts violent criminals who are lured by the huge profits that a black market creates.

Fortunately, though, much progress has been made in this regard in recent years. People can already legally purchase more-dangerous drugs (particularly when taken regularly over long periods) than illicit drugs—drugs such as alcohol and tobacco. And they don't need a doctor's prescription to buy and consume them. Forty-eight percent of Americans now live in jurisdictions where adults can purchase cannabis legally for recreational use and without a prescription.[87] More states and municipalities are allowing adults to buy hallucinogenic ("magic") mushrooms that contain psilocybin to use recreationally or therapeutically without a prescription. It should not be hard to imagine a world where adults can legally buy drugs that are less dangerous than alcohol and tobacco in a legal, competitive, and regulated market without needing a prescription; a market where wholesalers and retailers are held liable if they misinform or harm customers, and where consumers can access and exchange information comparing drugs and how to consume them safely—drugs including opioids, psychedelics, cocaine, and methamphetamine.

As when lawmakers ended alcohol prohibition nearly a century ago, they should recognize that drug prohibition has been a fatal mistake that has ended or ruined countless lives. It is long past the time to end the war on drugs.

CHAPTER 7

The War on Tobacco

The war on tobacco did not begin in the late 1960s. At the end of the 19th century, most people chewed tobacco or smoked cigars or pipes. The cigarette was an innovation that became popular after James Bonsack invented the automatic cigarette-rolling machine. A member of the Women's Christian Temperance Union, Lucy Page Gaston, founded the Chicago Anti-Cigarette League in 1890, contending that cigarette smoking was a dangerous habit that could entice young people and lead them to use alcohol and narcotics. Between 1890 and 1930, 15 states banned adults from selling, manufacturing, possessing, or using cigarettes.[1]

In the late 19th and early 20th century it was socially taboo for women to smoke, although many women smoked cigarettes in private. Some states and cities enacted laws that banned women from smoking. Journalist Cassandra Tate, in her book *Cigarette Wars*, writes, "In 1904, for example, a New York judge ordered a woman to jail for thirty days for smoking in front of her children. . . . Many companies, large and small, refused to hire cigarette smokers."[2]

New York City alderman Timothy Sullivan introduced a bill that barred the management of any public place from allowing women to smoke on their premises. The city council passed the so-called

Sullivan Ordinance unanimously, and it took effect in 1908. Katie Mulcahey was the ordinance's only victim. The city fined her five dollars, and she spent six months in jail for smoking in public. This sparked a fierce public debate over whether women should be free to smoke tobacco, and New York's mayor removed the Sullivan Ordinance after it was on the books for only two weeks.[3] Ironically, the ban emboldened proprietors of restaurants and similar businesses to invite women to smoke in their establishments.

States inconsistently enforced their anti-cigarette laws. Cigarette smoking grew more popular as soldiers returning from World War I embraced the practice and as women associated smoking with being independent.

By the end of the 1920s states had repealed their anti-smoking laws, as lawmakers decided it was easier to tax people who chose to smoke than to enforce prohibition. Kansas was the last of the 15 states to repeal cigarette prohibition in 1927.[4]

As the anti-smoking crusade petered out, smoking became fashionable, even de rigueur. Cigarette smoking played a significant role in many cinematic productions.[5] Examples include Hollywood classics such as Lauren Bacall and Humphrey Bogart in *To Have and Have Not* (1944); James Dean in *Rebel Without a Cause* (1955); and Anne Bancroft's Mrs. Robinson in *The Graduate* (1967). Cigarette advertisements featured celebrities. Some ads even featured doctors. The R. J. Reynolds Tobacco Company ran one ad that stated, "According to a nationwide survey: more doctors smoke Camels than any other cigarette" (see figure 7.1).[6]

By the late 1950s, as scientific evidence began linking tobacco smoking to lung cancer, cardiovascular disease, and other health problems, the anti-cigarette movement regained momentum. However, this time the crusade was based on, and enhanced by, scientific evidence rather than moralization and social taboo. The anti-cigarette campaign got a

FIGURE 7.1

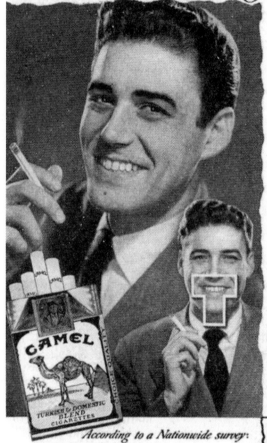

Source: The Center for the Study of Tobacco and Society.

big boost with the landmark surgeon general's report on smoking and health in 1964, which estimated a nine- to tenfold increase in the risk of lung cancer among smokers compared to nonsmokers.[7] As the scientific literature developed, federal and state lawmakers and public health institutions embarked on a campaign to educate people about the risks of smoking, ban public advertising of tobacco smoking products, place warning labels on cigarette packages, impose punitive "sin taxes" on tobacco smoking products, restrict marketing, and ban smoking in public places. These efforts combined to make cigarette smoking inconvenient, unfashionable, and, in some circles, socially unacceptable. As a result, by August 2023 Gallup reported that only 12 percent of American adults smoked cigarettes.[8] The CDC reported in November 2023 that only 1.1 percent of middle school students and 1.9 percent of high school students had smoked one or more cigarettes in the past 30 days.[9]

Externalities, Property Rights, and Consenting Adults

Laws banning smoking in restaurants, workplaces, and other privately owned venues where adults voluntarily interact infringe on adults' property rights and their right to informed consent. On the other hand, government restrictions on smoking in public areas where secondhand smoke poses a risk to others can be morally justifiable, based on the same principle that governments use to prohibit drunk driving: "The right to swing my fist ends where the other man's nose begins."[10] These are examples of what economists call "externalities": side effects or consequences of activities that affect other parties unintentionally. It is not morally justifiable for the government to ban individuals from smoking on their property. Nor is it justifiable to violate the rights of adults who socialize or conduct business on private property where the owners allow smoking and where adult participants willingly acknowledge the associated risks. Consumers wielding their market power will shape the policies of restaurant owners and other business owners regarding smoking on their premises. Likewise, the call for a smoke-free work environment will have an impact on the labor market and policies related to smoking in workplaces.

Courts have repeatedly found that government restrictions on most forms of tobacco advertising violate the free speech rights of tobacco makers and consumers.[11] However, in 1998, most tobacco companies entered into the Master Settlement Agreement with 52 state and territory attorneys general who sued them, accepting severe restrictions on advertising their products.[12]

Tobacco Prohibition Returns

In 2010, Bhutan became the first country to ban the sale of all tobacco products.[13] This generated a robust underground tobacco market, with many tobacco products coming in clandestinely from India. By 2017, Bhutan had a 24.6 percent smoking rate, the highest in Southeast Asia, and 29.3 percent of Bhutanese adolescents smoked.[14] In 2021, with smuggling of black-market tobacco rampant, and no significant drop in the smoking rate during the 11 years since the government had imposed the ban, the government ended tobacco prohibition, opting instead to tax and regulate tobacco sales.[15] Bhutanese policymakers also cited concerns that cross-border tobacco trafficking might increase the risk of spreading the COVID-19 virus amid the coronavirus pandemic.

Apparently, New Zealand lawmakers did not learn from Bhutan's experience. In 2022, the New Zealand government implemented legislation that banned the sale of tobacco products for everyone born after January 1, 2009—for life. At the same time, it cut back on the number of licensed tobacco retailers and ordered a gradual reduction in nicotine concentration in all tobacco products sold to existing legal customers. The goal was to create an entirely smoke-free generation beginning in 2027. This made New Zealand one of the most restrictive countries in the world concerning tobacco use. In November 2023, with less than 14 percent of New Zealanders smoking, the government scrapped the plan. A spokesperson for a tobacco ban advocacy group called the decision "a major loss for public health, and a huge win for the tobacco industry—whose profits will be boosted at the expense of Kiwi lives."[16] Just one month earlier, the UK government had announced plans to impose a phased-in tobacco ban like New Zealand's.[17] As of April 2024, Parliament was progressing the proposal through its legislative process.[18]

As of June 2024, Brookline, Massachusetts, is the only jurisdiction in the United States to have imposed a ban like New Zealand's.[19] Brookline bans the sale of tobacco to anyone born after 2000—for life. It doesn't take an entrepreneurial genius to figure out ways to make money legally selling cigarettes to adults from the other side of the Brookline town line.

In early 2023, California lawmakers considered making the Golden State the first in the country to enact New Zealand's tobacco prohibition model into law.[20] The bill failed to advance and didn't receive support from anti-smoking activists. A news report quoted Autumn Ogden-Smith, director of California state legislation for the American Cancer Society Cancer Action Network, saying, "This is not the time to tackle this. We're trying to do the clean-up on the flavored tobacco ban. We're having enforcement issues."[21]

Some jurisdictions have targeted flavored cigarettes especially aggressively. In 2019, Massachusetts lawmakers banned flavored tobacco, including menthol-flavored cigarettes, from the market. In 2020, California lawmakers followed suit. A 2023 study by the Reason Foundation concluded:

> In the 12-month period following the implementation of the comprehensive flavor ban in Massachusetts, the state sold 29.96 million fewer (22.24% less) cigarette packs compared to the prior year. However, a total of 33.3 million additional cigarette packs were

sold during the same post-ban period in the counties that bordered Massachusetts in the states of Connecticut (3.05 million additional packs), New Hampshire (25.84 million), New York (1.04 million), Rhode Island (6.01 million), and Vermont (1.21 million). Thus, considering the change in cigarette sales in the entire six-state region, there was a net increase of 7.21 million additional cigarette packs sold in the 12 months after the menthol cigarette ban in Massachusetts, a 1.28% increase in cigarette sales compared to the prior 12-month period before the ban.[22]

California is a much larger state than Massachusetts, and its largest cities are far from the state's borders, so it should not be as vulnerable to cross-border sales and smuggling. Yet a study by the Tax Foundation found that one year after the California ban went into effect, foreign and illicit tobacco sales spiked, including the number of duty-free cigarettes designated for export that found their way onto California's city streets. Smokers who prefer menthol and other flavored cigarettes are purchasing flavor and menthol inserts for cigarettes to work around the ban. While the state has lost tax revenue because people aren't buying menthol and flavored cigarettes legally, there has been no significant drop in the smoking rate.[23]

New York is also a large state. However, New York City's metropolitan area borders Connecticut and New Jersey, making cross-border sales relatively easy. New York City and New York State sought to subtly impose tobacco prohibition by imposing prohibitive cigarette excise taxes. This generated a robust black market in cigarettes, including people selling individual cigarettes, dubbed "loosies," on the street.[24] This black market increases the likelihood of confrontations between police and residents of minority communities, where selling individual cigarettes is popular. One infamous confrontation between New York City police and Eric Garner, who police suspected was selling loose cigarettes, ended in

Garner dying from a policeman's chokehold.[25] Jacob Sullum wrote
about the incident in *Reason*:

> By imposing excise taxes almost 20 times as high as those collected
> in a state that's a four-hour drive away, legislators invited the sort of
> entrepreneurial activity that got Garner into legal trouble. Some-
> thing like half of the cigarettes sold in New York City are smuggled
> from lower-tax jurisdictions. From Garner's perspective, he was per-
> forming a valued service for his neighbors by helping them avoid the
> country's heaviest cigarette taxes. From the city's perspective, he was
> depriving politicians of their cut, a Class A misdemeanor punishable
> by a maximum fine of $1,000 or up to a year in jail.[26]

According to a 2022 Tax Foundation study, New York has the highest cigarette smuggling rate in the country. California has the second
highest.[27]

Less than 2 percent of teens and adolescents reported having smoked
cigarettes within the past 30 days, as of November 2023.[28] According
to a 2022 report by the CDC, 60 percent of the vanishingly small number of teens who smoke choose nonmenthol cigarettes.[29] And a 2020
Reason Foundation study found that states with the highest menthol
consumption had the lowest youth smoking rates.[30]

The European Union banned menthol cigarettes in 2020. A recent
EU survey found that 40 percent of menthol smokers switched to nonmenthol and only 8 percent quit smoking. As in the United States,
European menthol smokers have come up with workarounds, such as
"mentholizing" recessed cigarette filters, using menthol flavor inserts,
or adding menthol to their tobacco.[31] However, 13 percent reported
getting menthol cigarettes from "other sources." A black market for
smuggled menthol cigarettes has emerged. A significant source is
Belarus, where menthol brands such as Minsk, Fest, and Queen find
their way into EU countries. The UK press reported that gangs smuggle

such "illicit whites" into the country, and people can buy them under the counter from British tobacconists for the right price.[32]

Worst of all, menthol bans can exacerbate racial and ethnic disparities in law enforcement and within the criminal justice system.[33] In public comments that I submitted to the FDA on its proposed menthol ban, I wrote the following:

> Prohibition fuels an underground market where peaceful voluntary transactions become crimes. It gives law enforcement another reason to interact with non-violent people who commit these victimless crimes. Like everyone else, police respond to incentives. They are rewarded by arrests and convictions. Low-level street dealers in illegal substances are "low-hanging fruit." They are much easier to find in dense inner cities, and less dangerous to confront than violent felons. Law enforcement tends to scour racial or ethnic minority communities for victimless crimes because they are "easy pickings." That's how we wind up with African Americans arrested for marijuana violations four times as often as whites, even though both ethnicities use marijuana roughly equally.
>
> And never forget Eric Garner. New York City's exorbitant taxes on cigarette packages generated an underground market in untaxed individual cigarettes, called "loosies." In 2014, police infamously encountered 43-year-old Eric Garner selling loosies on a street corner, and a policeman's chokehold led to his death as he repeated, "I can't breathe." This happened without a menthol ban.
>
> With menthol cigarettes more popular among Blacks and Hispanics, expect police to focus their attention on minority communities. The last thing this country needs is yet another reason for law enforcement to engage with minorities they suspect are committing the victimless crime of selling menthol cigarettes in the black market.[34]

After several civil rights groups, including the American Civil Liberties Union, expressed similar concerns about a blanket nationwide menthol ban exacerbating racial law enforcement disparities, in December 2023 President Biden announced a delay on the decision whether to ban menthol tobacco until March 2024.[35] In late April 2024, the Biden administration announced that it would further delay its decision. In a press release explaining the delay, Secretary of Health and Human Services Xavier Becerra announced that his department needs "significantly more time" to consider public comments and concerns about the proposed menthol ban.[36] The secretary did not give a target date for a decision.

Moreover, the health panic about menthol may be much ado about nothing. A 2011 prospective cohort study with more than 85,000 participants in 12 Southern states found that menthol smokers tended to smoke fewer cigarettes per day and that "menthol cigarettes are no more, and perhaps less harmful than non-menthol cigarettes."[37] Additionally, FDA researchers had reported in 2012 in the journal *Nicotine and Tobacco Research*, "We found evidence of lower lung cancer mortality risk among menthol smokers compared with nonmenthol smokers at ages 50 and over in the US population."[38] In April 2022, the FDA announced plans to ban all menthol cigarettes and cigars. Ironically, the announcement came in the wake of research published the same year showing that menthol smokers have no greater difficulty giving up smoking than nonmenthol smokers.[39] By early 2023, five states and 360 localities had enacted bans on flavored tobacco products, including menthol. Several other states are considering bans. In 2024, lawmakers in Hawaii, New York, Vermont, and Washington State were among those considering bans.[40]

Effectiveness aside, bans like the ones described above run roughshod over individuals' autonomy. Adults have the right to self-medicate and to consume whatever substances they wish—providing that they don't violate the rights of others—even when they risk their own health or life by doing so. Despite tobacco's health risks, many people derive pleasure from consuming tobacco and are willing to assume those risks. Policymakers should adhere to the principle articulated by John Stuart Mill that autonomous adults possess expertise in determining their own best interests, as they possess unique insights into their own well-being—priorities that others cannot comprehend.

It is appropriate for health care practitioners to inform their patients about the health hazards of tobacco products and advise against consuming them—in fact, it's the right thing to do. But clinicians cannot force patients to act based on the clinicians' perception of the patients' best interests. The government does not possess that right either.

CHAPTER 8

The Nascent War on Social Media "Addiction"

The internet is a new frontier for prohibitionists. Mental health experts, policymakers, and commentators express growing concern that social media platforms might be addictive and might contribute to mental health problems, particularly in adolescents and young adults.[1] At a September 2018 US Senate Intelligence Committee hearing on attempts by foreign adversaries to fabricate news stories and manipulate American public opinion, senators asked witnesses about the addictive power of social media.[2] Sen. Richard Burr (R-NC) expressed concern that media users, compelled by their addiction to face repeated exposure to propaganda and misinformation, might be increasingly vulnerable to manipulation.

Facebook CEO Mark Zuckerberg acknowledged the issue and expressed a commitment to addressing it. He told senators that his company was taking steps to give users more control over their experience and to promote healthier interactions on the platform. In an interview by the UK *Daily Telegraph*, Aaron Greenspan, one of the original creators of Facebook, claimed that the social media network is as addictive as tobacco and is costing lives.[3]

Fear about the risk of "internet addiction" or "social media addiction" (mental health experts use the terms interchangeably) is fueling lawmakers' interest in having the government restrict or block people from accessing the internet and social media sites, without any regard for adults' right to make their own risk-benefit assessments.[4]

While many behavioral health experts warn about social media addiction, researchers have not yet reached a consensus as to whether "excessive" time spent on the internet or interacting on social media constitutes addiction.[5] Policymakers often misuse the word "addiction": addiction refers to compulsively using a substance or engaging in an activity despite negative consequences. And the implications of whether social media addiction exists and how widespread it might be go beyond concerns about government intrusions on personal autonomy and control over behavioral choices in the name of public health.

The American Psychiatric Association's *Diagnostic and Statistical Manual of Mental Disorders* categorizes internet or social media addiction as a "condition for further study."[6] This is significant considering the strong economic incentives for the psychiatric profession to medicalize behavioral problems. However, a 2012 review of the scientific literature found that most reports are anecdotal and that peer-reviewed studies are scarce.[7] A 2017 follow-up study by the same research team found that the methodological problems persist.[8] And while some researchers link social media use with depression and even suicide, no causal relationship has been established.[9] Because of the controversy, while internet addiction treatment centers are springing up around the country, most health insurance plans will not pay for internet addiction treatment.[10] The cost of these programs can range from $3,000 to $45,000.[11]

Unlike the American Psychiatric Association, the World Health Organization recognizes "internet gaming disorder" in its 11th revision of the International Classification of Diseases, and China, South Korea, Japan, and other countries now consider internet addiction to be a mental health disorder.[12]

This is especially troubling in the case of a dictatorship such as China. The Chinese government officially recognized internet addiction disorder in 2008.[13] Since then, the Chinese government has limited the opening of new internet cafes and restricted the amount of time adolescents may spend at them. The government forces thousands of Chinese whom it labels "internet addicts" into psychiatric boot camps. It subjects them to forced medication and, sometimes, electroshock therapy.[14] This is reminiscent of how the Soviet Union used made-up mental health diagnoses to forcibly commit dissidents.[15]

China may present an extreme example, but the governments of many other countries—even some liberal democracies—have followed suit. In Japan, the Ministry of Health pays for "internet fasting camps," and the South Korean government blocks internet gaming sites for people under the age of 16 after midnight.[16] In December 2023 the European Parliament passed a resolution "targeting the addictive nature of digital platforms," greenlighting an initiative to devise new "consumer protection" regulations on scrolling and video autoplay.[17]

Anxieties about social media addiction may reach the level of today's panic over the opioid epidemic. People might demonize platforms such as X (formerly Twitter) and Facebook as purveyors of addictive content, portraying them in a manner similar to the way they perceive opioid pharmaceutical companies or Big Tobacco.

People wrongly see addiction as a disease in which individuals have no control over their choice to use the internet (or gamble or use alcohol or other drugs). The public more willingly accepts the government infringing on autonomy in such cases.

For example, suppose the government officially recognizes social media addiction as a disease. In that case, it may prompt lawmakers to pass laws or regulations requiring health plans to cover rehabilitation for this condition. This could lead to higher health insurance costs and increased public spending on programs such as Medicare and

Medicaid because lawmakers might feel motivated to allocate funding for the proliferation and expansion of social media treatment programs. This growing treatment industry could then become another special interest actively seeking a steady stream of government funds.[18]

Even worse, as the government becomes more involved in internet and social media activities, the risks to freedom of speech, freedom of the press, and freedom of association become more tangible. For example, in 2023, UK lawmakers passed a comprehensive internet safety law authorizing the government to punish digital platforms if they allow hate speech, information that the government decides is not age-appropriate, or information that can otherwise cause harm to children. German police have raided the homes of people across the country whom the government had charged with "hateful" postings over social media.[19] Fortunately, the US Constitution acts as a barrier to many laws like those implemented in other countries that involve the government in social media. American sensibilities also serve as a deterrent. The public is not currently in favor of such interventions— at least not yet.

It is not nitpicking to push back on talk about social media addiction. Journalists, commentators, and lawmakers should use terminology more accurately and precisely, and resist the temptation to confer legitimacy on an unproven addiction. This is not just a call for healthy skepticism—individual liberty and autonomy are at stake.

CHAPTER 9

What Is Harm Reduction?

Harm-reduction principles come easily to health care practitioners in affluent societies. Much of what we do every day is practice harm reduction.

Doctors routinely advise patients against making risky or unhealthy dietary, recreational, and other lifestyle choices. Patients seek care from us for conditions that might not need long-term medical treatment if they would abandon or modify their behavior. Some patients heed our advice, but others are unable or unwilling to do so. For example, a diet and exercise regimen can often correct high blood pressure, high cholesterol, or borderline diabetes. However, some patients find these regimens too challenging to follow. Some struggle to adjust their routine and need clinicians to supplement their efforts with medication. Some patients don't want to give up the pleasures or other positive values they derive from their routines—they weigh the tradeoffs and accept the risk.

When doctors prescribe medication to treat patients' blood pressure, high cholesterol, or borderline diabetes, they engage in harm reduction. They don't endorse their patients' choices. They warn them of the hazards. Instead, they do what they can to reduce the harmful effects that result.

Harm reduction is realistic and nonjudgmental. Clinicians don't attach conditions when they engage in harm reduction. They don't refuse to treat patients unless they first change their behavior. Doctors don't insist that their patients agree in writing to adopt a diet and exercise plan before they prescribe a GLP-1 drug to treat patients' obesity (such as Ozempic or Wegovy, which stimulate the body to produce insulin and reduce appetite and food cravings), and then hold them to the contract. They don't refuse to prescribe aerosol nebulizers or oxygen to smokers who develop chronic lung disease unless the patients abstain from smoking. This nonjudgmental approach to patients and respect for their autonomy is the essence of harm reduction.

Yet for many lawmakers and policymakers who view some behaviors as immoral or taboo, the nonjudgmental aspect of harm reduction has a negative connotation. The term puts off many policymakers, who equate harm reduction with enabling people to use some drugs or engage in certain activities that the policymakers disapprove of.[1]

The term "harm reduction" originated in the 1980s in Liverpool, England, as an epidemic of HIV/AIDS (a result of intravenous drug users sharing contaminated needles) spread across Britain. The epidemic had already spread to Edinburgh, Scotland. Authorities there responded by doubling down on law enforcement, arresting drug dealers, banning needle sales, and closing methadone treatment centers. The epidemic had not yet reached Liverpool, where local activists, most notably Russell Newcombe, Alan Parry, and a physician named John Marks (who had already been prescribing heroin—which is legal, but strictly regulated in the UK—to addicted patients so they wouldn't seek it in the black market), organized volunteers to distribute clean needles to drug users and educate users on how to sterilize their equipment. They engaged in outreach to drug users and sex workers (many of whom also used drugs), two of the groups most vulnerable to HIV/AIDS. As a result, Liverpool averted the devastation that HIV/AIDS brought to Edinburgh.[2]

Newcombe coined the term "harm reduction" in a 1987 article, "High Time for Harm Reduction."[3] The activists founded a journal, organized conferences, and drew attention from policymakers around world, including in the United States. In an August 2022 interview, harm-reduction historian Maia Szalavitz said that Margaret Thatcher, who was the UK's conservative prime minister at the time, was no fan of illicit drug use yet she saw the logic and success of the Liverpool project and concluded that "HIV is a bigger threat than drugs; proceed."[4]

Today, we use harm reduction in myriad contexts. Partiers who intend to consume large quantities of alcohol and agree on a designated driver are engaging in harm reduction. Other examples of harm reduction include seat belts in vehicles, bicycle helmets, football helmets, batting helmets, hard hats, and respiratory masks for painters. Policymakers make no efforts to block these forms of harm reduction—they even encourage it.

Policymakers have no aversion to doctors prescribing medications to their patients to reduce harm from some of their lifestyle choices, such as those related to diet and exercise. However, the government impedes patients from accessing some forms of harm reduction by determining which medications they can buy legally and by often requiring them to get prescriptions from clinicians in order to buy them.

Yet policymakers strike a different chord when it comes to using harm-reduction strategies for some risky behaviors, such as smoking tobacco and consuming some drugs.

Federal and state drug paraphernalia laws make it illegal to manufacture, sell, distribute, possess, or use items such as clean needles and syringes, fentanyl test strips, and other drug-testing equipment.[5] In many states, harm-reduction organizations—or just compassionate individuals—risk arrest for handing fentanyl test strips to people they know who consume illicit drugs.[6] Recently, some states have exempted fentanyl test strips from their list of outlawed paraphernalia.[7] As prohibition fuels drug cartels to develop newer and more potent forms of illicit drugs, drug device manufacturers have developed testing equipment to check for them. Where states have only exempted fentanyl test strips from the list of banned testing equipment, lawmakers will need to pass additional legislation to exempt them from any ban—unless they make things easier by exempting all testing equipment.[8]

A federal law, 21 U.S.C. Section 856, called the "crack house" statute, makes it a felony to "knowingly open, lease, rent, use, or maintain any place . . . for the purpose of manufacturing, distributing, or using any controlled substance."[9] This law bars harm-reduction organizations from establishing overdose prevention centers (OPCs), a proven harm-reduction strategy that started in Switzerland in 1986 and has been saving lives in 148 locations and 16 countries for decades.[10] New York City's two OPCs reported reversing more than 1,000 overdoses slightly more than one year after they opened. In Canada, researchers reported in The Lancet in early 2024 that OPCs averted two overdose fatalities per 100,000 people in neighborhoods surrounding OPCs in Toronto in 2019.[11]

Federal and state laws impose barriers on patients getting access to methadone treatment for opioid addiction or dependency.[12] Until recently, federal laws restricted access to buprenorphine, another medication used for opioid use disorder.[13]

Federal and state governments block tobacco smokers' access to proven harm-reduction tools such as nicotine-containing e-cigarettes, particularly flavored ones, which surveys show that smokers prefer to use to help them quit.[14] More recently, federal lawmakers have called on federal agencies to restrict access to tobacco-free nicotine pouches, a form of nicotine replacement therapy that can help many smokers give up the habit.[15]

Governments apply a double standard toward harm reduction. They leave people relatively free to access harm-reduction strategies when they engage in behavior or consume substances that governments approve of. They block access to harm reduction for those who consume substances or engage in behaviors of which governments disapprove.

The government's war on some drugs assaults autonomy on two fronts: it infringes on people's right to put into their bodies whatever substances they desire and it tramples on their right to reduce the risk of doing so.

CHAPTER 10

Tobacco Harm Reduction

In the 1950s, scientific evidence of tobacco's harms emerged to spark the modern anti-smoking movement. Research demonstrated that the tar, carbon monoxide, and toxic chemicals in the tobacco leaf are the main culprits responsible for causing cancers, cardiovascular disease, and lung problems.[1] America's love/hate relationship with tobacco dates to the late 19th century, when members of the Women's Christian Temperance Movement founded the Anti-Cigarette League of America in 1890.[2] By the late 1950s, the anti-smoking movement had science instead of moralizing to back it up.

Anti-smoking activists should claim success. In 2023, adult tobacco smoking reached a historic low of 11 percent of adults, down from 42 percent in the 1960s.[3] Less than 1 percent of teens today light up daily.[4] However, instead of acknowledging success, numerous anti-smoking activists are now adopting inconsistent and seemingly contradictory stances on how to reduce the harms of tobacco use.[5] In the process, they threaten adults' right to seek harm-reduction strategies.

Nicotine Replacement Therapy

According to a 2016 FDA survey, most lay people think that nicotine, a compound found in tobacco, is dangerous and causes cancer.[6]

However, while nicotine is the component of tobacco smoke to which people become addicted, the substance is relatively harmless. Britain's Royal Society for Public Health claims that nicotine is "no more harmful to health than caffeine."[7] As the UK's *NHS Inform* website states, "Although nicotine is a very addictive substance, it is relatively harmless. It's the carbon monoxide, tar and other toxic chemicals in tobacco smoke that'll cause serious damage to your health. Clear forms of nicotine . . . don't have any additives or toxic chemicals and are proven to be safe and effective."[8]

Nicotine is present in our diet in small doses. For example, tomatoes, potatoes, and eggplants are good sources of nicotine. A tobacco cigarette contains roughly 12 milligrams of nicotine (approximately 18 times the 675 nanograms of nicotine found in a potato), but smokers absorb less than 2 milligrams of nicotine per cigarette.[9] While most people smoke more than one cigarette in a day, it's the harmful chemicals in cigarette smoke, not the nicotine alone, that cause most of the health risks associated with smoking.

Nicotine, like caffeine, stimulates and enhances concentration. Unlike caffeine, nicotine increases beta-endorphins, which helps relieve anxiety. This may explain why people say "I need a cigarette" to calm down under stress. Also, like caffeine, nicotine can be addictive.[10] However, if people use tobacco as their nicotine delivery system, they continuously expose themselves to tobacco's harmful compounds. Consuming nicotine long-term can cause high blood pressure and may contribute to blood vessel narrowing. Prolonged caffeine consumption can cause ulcers, irregular heartbeat, tremors, and insomnia.

Some research suggests that nicotine may help treat Parkinson's disease.[11] There is also evidence that nicotine may help treat depression, Tourette syndrome, Alzheimer's disease, and schizophrenia.[12] Many tobacco smokers—whether they are addicted to nicotine or not, either consciously or unconsciously—are using cigarettes or cigars to get nicotine. Some may be self-medicating. Nicotine replacement therapy (NRT) is a harm-reduction strategy that provides people with safer ways to get their nicotine.

Nicotine gum and nicotine patches are examples of NRT. They provide alternative, safer ways for people to get their nicotine. Varenicline is a different kind of smoking cessation aid: it's a pill that works by blocking nicotine receptors in the brain so that users cannot experience nicotine's desirable effects. People take varenicline to abstain from nicotine as opposed to consuming it more safely.

For many people, NRT works better when it more closely mimics smoking. For example, nicotine e-cigarettes allow consumers to inhale and exhale a vapor ("vaping") containing nicotine while avoiding the carcinogens and toxic chemicals of tobacco smoke. A 2019 randomized trial reported in the *New England Journal of Medicine* found nicotine e-cigarettes to be superior to other forms of nicotine replacement therapy for reducing or quitting smoking.[13] A 2022 Cochrane systematic review found "high certainty evidence" that e-cigarettes are superior to other forms of NRT for smoking cessation.[14] Researchers reporting in *The Lancet* in 2023 on a naturalistic randomized controlled clinical trial found that "unguided" e-cigarette uptake helped tobacco smokers quit.[15] A Swiss study published in the *New England Journal of Medicine* in 2024 concluded, "The addition of e-cigarettes to standard smoking-cessation counseling resulted in greater abstinence from tobacco use among smokers than smoking-cessation counseling alone."[16]

At the federal level, Congress has made it illegal for retailers to sell e-cigarettes to anyone under the age of 21, out of concerns that teen vaping of nicotine e-cigarettes might be a gateway to tobacco smoking.[17] Yet researchers at Brown and Harvard Universities, using data from 2008 to 2018, reported, "E-cigarette use is largely concentrated among youth who share characteristics with smokers of the pre-vaping era, suggesting e-cigarettes may have replaced cigarette smoking." The authors state in the study's abstract:

> Among non-smoking youth, vaping is largely concentrated among those who would likely have smoked prior to the introduction of e-cigarettes, and the introduction of e-cigarettes has coincided with an acceleration in the decline in youth smoking rates. E-cigarettes may be an important tool for population-level harm reduction, even considering their impact on youth.[18]

One of the study's authors, Natasha Sokol, told an interviewer, "The decline in youth smoking really accelerated after the availability of e-cigarettes."[19] Teen e-cigarette use has been declining as well, with only 10 percent of high schoolers in 2023 reporting having vaped in the last 30 days.[20]

Concern about teen vaping has led many states to ban adults from obtaining flavored e-cigarettes.[21] The FDA continues to curtail companies from marketing flavored e-cigarettes.[22] While flavored e-cigarettes are popular among teens, they are also the choice of 90 percent of adult tobacco smokers who use e-cigarettes to quit smoking.[23] Surveys repeatedly show that anywhere from 92 to 94 percent of former smokers who switched to vaping preferred the fruit-, candy-, or menthol-flavored varieties.[24]

Policymakers do not only target flavored e-cigarettes. The FDA is blocking adults from obtaining many unflavored nicotine e-cigarettes as well.[25] Yet flavored and unflavored e-cigarettes from China and other countries are available for sale in a flourishing black market, where young and old alike can buy products of uncertain quality.[26]

Federal and state governments are waging an indefensible cold war on e-cigarette users. These governments are flouting adults' autonomy. Laws should not prohibit adults from consuming substances or

engaging in activities simply because they are dangerous or harmful if children do them. There is also evidence that policies against
e-cigarettes are counterproductive, as they are making many adults
who had switched from smoking to vaping go back to smoking.[27]

Heated Tobacco Products

Heated tobacco devices deliver nicotine using a device that resembles an
e-cigarette. However, e-cigarettes don't use tobacco. E-cigarettes heat
liquid nicotine from 300°F to 600°F to produce a nicotine-containing
vapor. Cigarettes burn tobacco to a temperature of 1300°F, delivering
the nicotine in a smoke that contains numerous harmful chemicals.
Heated tobacco devices don't burn the tobacco but instead heat it to
600°F to deliver nicotine to the user in an aerosol containing a much
lower concentration of carcinogens and other harmful compounds
than is found in tobacco smoke.[28]

Heated tobacco devices enable people to enjoy tobacco and nicotine
in a less harmful form, which makes them a worthwhile component
of the tobacco harm-reduction arsenal. Heated tobacco products are
popular in Europe and Japan, but the FDA has slowed their arrival in
the United States.[29] Surveys suggest that most people who consume
heated tobacco products don't do so to quit smoking but instead see
heated tobacco as a safer way to enjoy tobacco.[30] Data from Japan and
elsewhere suggest that heated tobacco products drive down cigarette
sales and don't appeal to youth.[31]

In late 2022, the European Union banned residents from purchasing flavored heated tobacco products.[32] While the US government
has not yet explicitly banned its residents from obtaining flavored
heated tobacco products, as of January 2023 the FDA has only permitted adults to buy a handful of tobacco-flavored heated tobacco
products.[33]

Snus

For anti-smoking crusaders who are uncomfortable with the idea of people inhaling smoke, aerosol, or vapor to get their nicotine, there is an alternative form of NRT called *snus*, which is popular in Sweden. Swedes developed snus in the 17th century. It is a moistened tobacco product that people place between the lip and gum, much like smoke-less tobacco, where it slowly releases nicotine. However, the tobacco is steam-pasteurized, which gives it a lower concentration of the compounds in smokeless or chewing tobacco that can cause oral and throat cancer. Also, unlike smokeless tobacco or chewing tobacco, users don't need to spit out the saliva, which they can swallow instead, when they are done sucking or chewing the tobacco. Consumers can buy it loose in small canisters or in packets resembling tea bags. Snus became so popular in Sweden that it led to the creation of a tobacco-growing industry in the country.[34]

Inexplicably, while heated tobacco products and chewing tobacco are permissible, the European Union bans adults from obtaining snus everywhere except in Sweden.[35] Australia and New Zealand don't allow adults to obtain snus in their countries, nor does the United Kingdom. Meanwhile, Canada, Norway, Switzerland, and the United States respect adults' right to obtain and consume snus.

In Sweden, for the past 30 years, snus has been more popular than smoking among men. Over the same period, smoking in Norway has also decreased, while consuming snus has increased.[36] A recent study revealed that Sweden has the lowest daily cigarette use rate, the lowest tobacco-related mortality rate, and the lowest male lung cancer rate in the European Union.[37]

It is incoherent for governments to block adults from this safer alternative to traditional tobacco as a nicotine delivery system.

Nicotine Pouches

Nicotine pouches should hit the sweet spot for anti-smoking activists who have an aversion to harm-reduction strategies that either mimic smoking behavior, such as e-cigarettes, or those that use the tobacco plant. Nicotine pouches are a tobacco-free nicotine delivery system. They usually come in flavors. Brands include Zyn, On!, and Velo. Like snus, they work by users placing them between the lips and gums, where they slowly release nicotine.

In early 2023, Senate Majority Leader Chuck Schumer (D-NY) held a press conference expressing alarm that young "influencers" were using Zyn brand nicotine pouches on social media platforms such as TikTok. He called on the FDA to investigate the product for health concerns and on the Federal Trade Commission to investigate the manufacturer's marketing methods.[38] Schumer used words including "dangerous," "highly addictive," and "packed with health problems" to describe the Zyn brand nicotine pouches and warned that they are a danger to teens. He also invited a medical doctor to the podium to tell the audience that nicotine may cause harm to developing brains. Guy Bentley, a policy analyst at Reason Foundation, described Schumer's campaign as "severely misguided" and claimed that Schumer was trying to "whip up a moral panic against products that save lives."[39]

The Centers for Disease Control and Prevention reported in November 2023 that only 1.5 percent of middle school and high school students use nicotine pouches.[40] While there is indeed evidence suggesting that regular nicotine consumption might cause harm to the developing brain, most of the evidence is based on observational studies or animal experiments.[41] For perspective, regular use of caffeine or alcohol can also harm the developing brain, and pediatricians advise parents not to let their children drink coffee.[42] As with alcohol, e-cigarettes, and snus, in the United States people must be aged 21 and over to buy nicotine pouches.

However, by stoking public fears this way, Schumer might lead the public and their political representatives to make poor policy choices. And he is not alone. The Truth Initiative, which describes itself as "America's largest nonprofit public health organization dedicated to a future free from lifelong [addiction]," warns people on its website against using Zyn and other nicotine pouches and provides advice on how they can quit.[43]

Why this aversion to a drug that is no more harmful than caffeine? Why aren't organizations breathlessly arranging anti-coffee and anti-caffeine campaigns?

As ever-decreasing numbers of adults and youth take up tobacco smoking, anti-smoking activists appear to be targeting any substance or activity that, in any way, connects their thoughts to tobacco smoking.[44] Like the people the FDA surveyed in 2016 who believe that nicotine causes cancer, many anti-smoking activists seem to equate nicotine with tobacco's harms. How else to explain this baseless and irrational fear of nicotine, this nicotinophobia?[45]

Nicotinophobia jeopardizes the right of autonomous adults to consume tobacco-free nicotine and appreciate nicotine's benefits while acknowledging its associated risks.

CHAPTER 11

Harm-Reduction Strategies for People Who Use Illicit Drugs

Many adults who choose to consume illicit drugs realize they are risking harm. They perform a risk-benefit analysis and conclude that the benefits—either pleasure or physical or psychic pain relief—outweigh the risks. Ironically, many of the harms that come from using illicit drugs directly result from the drugs being illegal. If governments ended their war on these drugs, it would become much safer for people to consume them.

Like alcohol and most drugs, it can be lethal to consume too high of a dose of opioids. Unlike the legal drug alcohol, however, opioids don't cause cirrhosis of the liver, pancreatitis, stomach or esophageal cancer, cardiomyopathy, or encephalopathy. Long-term use of opioids can cause constipation, and there is evidence that it can affect testosterone and estrogen levels, which can lead to osteoporosis.[1] When adults purchase liquor from a legal dealer, the label on the bottle displays the alcohol percentage of this drug. Consumers need not worry that the makers of the alcoholic beverage might have laced it with another drug or allowed impurities to contaminate it. They can more safely consume the drug when they know its potency and purity.

However, people who purchase illicit drugs from underground dealers can never be sure of a drug's dose or purity—or even if it is the drug

they think they are buying. This increases the risk that they will overdose either from the drug they are buying or a contaminant. There are
myriad press reports about people who died from fentanyl overdoses
when they purchased and consumed what they thought was cocaine or
methamphetamine or a prescription pain pill.[2]

Harm-reduction strategies for illicit drug users aim to mitigate the
harmful effects of drug prohibition. By infringing on adults' right to
self-medicate, governments make self-medication more dangerous than
it would otherwise be. By enforcing drug prohibition, governments
incentivize drug trafficking organizations to develop more potent,
deadly, and easy-to-conceal drugs (see "The Iron Law of Prohibition,"
chapter 6). Governments further compound the harm by barring people from accessing tools to make self-medication less harmful.

Naloxone

The opioid overdose antidote naloxone, which the FDA approved for
use in 1971, works by binding to opioid receptors and displacing opioids that are already bound to those receptors. It is an effective remedy
that lay people can safely administer with minimal training to overdose victims by using a nasal spray, an intramuscular auto-injector, or
intravenously. It can reverse the respiratory depression caused by an
opioid overdose within 2 to 8 minutes, and its effects last about 30 to
90 minutes.[3]

Naloxone is one of the most basic and effective harm-reduction
tools. It has few to no side effects if opioids are not present in the
patient's body. In an opioid-dependent user, however, it can precipitate
withdrawal symptoms by pushing off opioid molecules that are bound
to a patient's receptors and blocking them from returning. Naloxone
is nevertheless so effective at reducing deaths from overdose that the
World Health Organization includes the drug on its list of essential
medicines for the treatment of opioid dependence.[4]

Up until 2023, the FDA barred people from obtaining naloxone without a permission slip from a government-licensed gatekeeper.[5] Most state policymakers have developed workarounds by authorizing pharmacists to prescribe naloxone or by permitting licensed physicians to issue standing orders to pharmacists throughout the state to dispense naloxone to patients under the physician's name.

Ironically, in 2016, the FDA announced that it believed it was probably appropriate to reclassify naloxone as an over-the-counter drug and asked manufacturers to request that the agency consider reclassifying it. The naloxone manufacturers did not respond with reclassification requests. The FDA commissioner had the authority to act without any request but continued deferring to the drug makers.[6] The governments of Australia, Belgium, Croatia, Denmark, Estonia, France, Germany, Italy, Malta, Norway, Spain, and Sweden had removed barriers to over-the-counter access to naloxone years earlier.[7]

Finally, the FDA announced in February 2023 that it would permit adults to purchase nasal spray versions of naloxone, and, in March 2023, it permitted adults to purchase Narcan brand nasal spray, over the counter without a prescription. However, non-nasal spray forms of naloxone, which are less expensive than the nasal spray, remain prescription-only.[8] Harm-reduction organizations and people who use opioids must still rely on the workarounds to access the cheaper forms of naloxone. The government should remove the barriers to patients obtaining all remaining forms of naloxone over the counter.

Drug Paraphernalia Laws

In 1979, President Jimmy Carter asked the Drug Enforcement Administration to develop model legislation for states to enact drug paraphernalia laws.[9] By 1981, 20 states had enacted drug paraphernalia laws based on the DEA's model act. By 2023, every state except Alaska had enacted drug paraphernalia laws.[10] However, in May 2023, Minnesota repealed its drug paraphernalia laws.[11]

State-level drug paraphernalia laws prevent individuals from protecting themselves against many of the risks of using drugs obtained on the black market. Some paraphernalia laws deny drug users access to fentanyl test strips, which are a vital means of screening drugs for contamination with fentanyl, the dangerous opioid that is responsible for the majority of opioid-related overdose deaths. Some paraphernalia laws restrict people from purchasing or possessing clean needles and syringes, thus increasing their risk of infection from sharing and reusing those items.

Drug paraphernalia laws also threaten to punish nonusers who engage in harm reduction. People risk incarceration if they give out or obtain clean needles and syringes, test strips, or materials to clean drug-use equipment. Paraphernalia laws prevent private organizations from creating syringe services programs (SSPs), previously known as needle exchange programs. These programs reduce the spread of HIV, hepatitis, and other blood-borne infectious diseases, as well as soft tissue infections, and they stopped an outbreak of HIV in intravenous drug users in Scott County, Indiana, in 2014.[12] Research shows that they reduced injection-risk behavior in Florida.[13] As of September 2022, the California Department of Health reported that it had 65 SSPs in 33 counties, which played a "central role in steeply reducing HIV transmission in California, reducing hepatitis B and C virus transmission, and preventing skin and soft tissue infections among people who use drugs."[14] More recently, they have proven helpful in reducing drug overdoses by distributing fentanyl test strips and naloxone along with clean syringes.[15]

Federal and state paraphernalia laws prohibit or severely restrict access to equipment that can help people use drugs more safely. Federal laws prohibit transporting drug paraphernalia across state lines, whereas state laws focus on intrastate trafficking. Federal and state statutes vary in how and what they define as paraphernalia. Both federal and state paraphernalia laws obstruct private harm-reduction organizations that seek to save lives, but state paraphernalia laws have a more direct and deleterious effect on harm reduction.

Under the federal drug paraphernalia section of the Controlled Substances Act, it is illegal to sell, transport through the mail, import, export, or transport across state lines "any equipment, product or material of any kind which is primarily intended or designed for use in manufacturing, compounding, converting, concealing, producing, processing, preparing, injecting, ingesting, inhaling, or otherwise introducing into the human body a controlled substance." Examples include pill presses, glass and metal pipes used to smoke crack cocaine and methamphetamine, specialized glass products, scales, cone-shaped marijuana/hash pipes called "chillums," and even miniature spoons.[16] Compounding pharmacies must register pill presses and other drug-making and testing equipment with the DEA and keep detailed records of all transactions for two years.[17]

States vary in what they define as drug paraphernalia. For example, Arizona prohibits possession "with intent to use, drug paraphernalia to plant, propagate, cultivate, grow, harvest, manufacture, compound, convert, produce, process, prepare, test, analyze, pack, repack, store, contain, conceal, inject, ingest, inhale or otherwise introduce into the human body a drug in violation of this chapter."[18] Illinois law specifies as prohibited paraphernalia "testing equipment intended to be used unlawfully in a private home for identifying or in analyzing the strength, effectiveness, or purity of controlled substances."[19]

For decades, harm-reduction organizations have operated drug-checking centers at music and dance festivals and parties. Organizations such as DanceSafe analyze users' drug samples with more sophisticated equipment than test strips while protecting their anonymity.

Drug-checking centers have been commonplace in the Netherlands, Austria, and much of Europe for decades, and public health authorities in Australia and New Zealand have recently begun promoting them.[20] Studies have shown that drug-checking centers provide safer venues for festival goers.[21] In one study, one in five specimens submitted by UK festival goers was "not as sold or acquired," and the testing organization informed the users before they consumed them.[22] Yet in many states drug paraphernalia laws make drug-checking centers illegal or else their legal status is unclear.[23]

Many states consider fentanyl test strips to be drug paraphernalia and ban them because individuals use them to test or analyze illicit drugs. As a result, people end up overdosing because the ban prevents them from determining what would be a nonlethal dose.[24]

Over the past few years, many states have amended their drug paraphernalia laws to exclude fentanyl test strips. In those states, people who distribute fentanyl test strips to people who use illicit drugs are no longer risking arrest for criminal conduct.[25]

However, because of the iron law of prohibition—the harder the law enforcement, the harder the drug—drug traffickers added the veterinary tranquilizer xylazine to fentanyl, creating what users call "tranq." The DEA reported finding xylazine in 23 percent of the fentanyl powder and fentanyl pills it seized in 2022.[26] Fortunately, the company that manufactures fentanyl test strips now makes xylazine test strips.[27] And as new synthetic opioids called nitazenes have emerged to cause a potential new wave of overdose deaths, hopefully some company will develop nitazene test strips.

Yet most states have not amended their paraphernalia laws to exempt xylazine test strips, and lawmakers will need to pass new legislation for that to happen. Here's a suggestion for lawmakers: exempt *all* drug-testing equipment from drug paraphernalia laws.[28] However, this would be a second-best option. The best option is to repeal paraphernalia laws altogether.

Federal law does not interfere with states operating or permitting privately run SSPs. However, many state drug paraphernalia laws prohibit these services. Some states carve out exceptions for SSPs in their drug paraphernalia laws, yet these exceptions often include restrictions on the number of SSPs that are allowed, restrictions on the entities that may operate them, and onerous conditions that they must meet.[29]

Decades of evidence on SSPs show that they reduce drug overdoses and the spread of HIV, hepatitis, and other blood-borne infectious diseases. They also promote and facilitate treatment and rehabilitation of participants who suffer from substance use disorder.[30] These programs distribute clean needles and syringes to intravenous drug users. Many programs also distribute fentanyl test strips along with bleach and other materials to clean syringes and needles. Most distribute naloxone. Some offer HIV and hepatitis blood tests and refer those who test positive for medical treatment.

The Centers for Disease Control and Prevention endorses and promotes SSPs with guidance and, in some cases, provides financial assistance to local jurisdictions for these facilities.[31] The World Health Organization, the American Medical Association, the American Public Health Association, the American Society of Addiction Medicine, and the American Psychiatric Association all support and encourage SSPs. The Substance Abuse and Mental Health Services Administration and the National Academies of Sciences, Engineering, and Medicine also endorse SSPs.

The empirical evidence shows that SSPs save lives by reducing the spread of deadly and infectious diseases without increasing illicit drug use or crime.[32] Furthermore, SSPs reduce disease among intravenous drug users' intimate contacts who are not engaging in illicit drug use and they also might possibly reduce disease spread to first responders.

With the advent of state laws facilitating the wider distribution of fentanyl test strips and naloxone, studies suggest that SSPs might reduce overdose deaths as well.[33]

States that clarify or modify their paraphernalia laws to legally authorize SSPs impose various restrictions on their structure and operation, as well as on state-level funding opportunities. Restrictions on how SSPs operate limit their scope, hamper their success, and work against the goal of reducing the spread of disease.

In Alaska, which has no statewide drug paraphernalia laws on the books, charitable and other nongovernmental organizations can implement SSPs and other harm-reduction strategies. In 2023, Minnesota became the first state to emulate Alaska. Until federal and state drug prohibition ends, the best way to reduce the risks of harm from using drugs obtained in the illegal market is for states to emulate Alaska and Minnesota by repealing their drug paraphernalia laws.

Eliminating state drug paraphernalia laws will let SSPs and other evidence-based harm-reduction strategies work to their full potential and, more importantly, will allow drug users to reduce harm to themselves.

Overdose Prevention Centers

Although SSPs can reduce the risk of overdose by distributing fentanyl test strips and naloxone, they are likely to be less effective if people use drugs in unsupervised settings. For example, users who inject when they are alone may have difficulty using naloxone to reverse an overdose.

During alcohol prohibition, speakeasies provided a secret and relatively safe place to consume an illegal drug. Overdose prevention centers (OPCs) got their start as the speakeasies of today's war on drugs. Harm-reduction pioneers initially called them "safe consumption sites." Some European jurisdictions call them "drug consumption rooms." The world's first professionally staffed—yet illegal—consumption room opened in Rotterdam, the Netherlands, in the early 1970s. In 1986, the illegal consumption site Contact Netz began operating in a café in Bern, Switzerland. The Swiss government eventually removed legal obstacles to Contact Netz serving clients who were older than age 18, making it the first legal overdose prevention center in the world. The Dutch government officially approved such centers in 1996.[34]

Overdose prevention centers have more ambitious goals than SSPs. They furnish people who use drugs with sterile syringes and needles. They allow drug users to inject illicitly obtained drugs in a clean, indoor clinical setting, out of public view, where users are free from harassment and the risks of theft and physical or sexual assault. On-site health care professionals have naloxone available to treat overdoses and can refer patients for medical treatment and rehabilitation. The centers provide equipment for drug users to test their drugs for fentanyl and other contaminants. Drug users must return syringes after using them to prevent passing or selling used needles and syringes to others.

In recent years, many drug users in the United States have switched from injecting to inhaling (snorting or smoking) drugs, as in much of the rest of the world.[35] With inhalation, drug users can better adjust the amount of drug they consume to reach the desired effect and avoid taking too large a dose, as often happens when injecting. OPCs often provide clean and safe inhalation devices to those clients and most facilities require users to spend time in "chill-out rooms" to allow the drug's initial effects to subside so the user is less impaired when leaving the site. OPCs also may provide showers and other facilities and connect users to social services.[36] Many clients respond to the nonjudgmental, caring atmosphere of safe consumption sites by seeking treatment and other social services.[37]

Today, 148 sanctioned OPCs operate in 16 countries and 92 communities around the world. Before October 2024, no OPC had ever reported a client dying from an overdose.[38] Sadly, staff at a London, Ontario, OPC experienced their first overdose fatality in early October 2024 after being unable to resuscitate an overdose victim.[39] Most OPCs are closely monitored by government agencies, which makes it difficult for them to conceal overdoses. Even if states repeal their drug paraphernalia laws and explicitly permit OPCs, a federal statute, 21 USC Section 856, colloquially known as the "crack house statute," makes it illegal for an establishment to permit people to use federally banned substances on its premises and so it blocks harm-reduction organizations from opening.[40]

New York City sanctioned two OPCs, one in East Harlem and one in Washington Heights, at the end of November 2021. A nonprofit harm-reduction organization, OnPointNYC, operates both in defiance of federal law. By the summer of 2023 OnPointNYC reported that it had reversed more than 1,000 overdoses.[41] The federal government had not acted against the OPCs as of late 2024.

In July 2021, Rhode Island governor Dan McKee signed into law a bill that defies the crack house statute by permitting privately funded harm-reduction organizations to operate OPCs if they are sanctioned by local public health authorities and if they continuously provide those authorities with outcomes data.[42] A partnership of two harm-reduction organizations called Project Weber/RENEW opened the Ocean State's first sanctioned OPC in Providence in December of 2024.[43] By early 2024 there were signs that Minnesota and Massachusetts might also defy federal law and permit harm-reduction organizations to operate OPCs.

Many state and federal lawmakers want to deny people the right to use drugs that the government doesn't approve of in safer environments, where they can mitigate some of the dangers to which drug prohibition would otherwise expose them. These lawmakers oppose efforts to repeal the crack house statute or at least amend the law so that harm-reduction organizations can operate OPCs and save lives. Many lawmakers oppose OPCs because they believe OPCs enable people to use government-banned drugs.[44] However, banning OPCs places people who use prohibited drugs, including chemically dependent addicts, in the difficult position of choosing between abstaining or risking death.

Treating Substance Use Disorder

Removing barriers to treatment is another type of harm reduction. If the government removed barriers to treating people with substance use disorders, more people would get treatment, which would help reduce the number of people seeking drugs in the black market. There are no effective medicine-assisted treatments for people who are dependent on or addicted to stimulants such as methamphetamine or cocaine. However, there are medications that effectively treat people with opioid use disorder (OUD).

Opioid addiction and opioid dependency are two distinct subsets of OUD. Dependency refers to the physiologic adaptation to the drug; abrupt cessation can cause a physical withdrawal reaction. Addiction is a behavioral disorder characterized by compulsive use despite negative consequences. People with addiction still feel compelled to use opioids even when they are no longer physically dependent on them.[45]

Much evidence confirms that long-term treatment with the opioid agonists methadone and buprenorphine is the most effective treatment for OUD. The *Merriam-Webster* dictionary defines an agonist as "a chemical substance capable of combining with a specific receptor on a cell and initiating the same reaction or activity typically produced by the binding endogenous (self-generated) substance."[46] These medications work to stabilize the lives of people with OUD by eliminating the fear of painful withdrawal symptoms *without* impairing their cognitive faculties. This reduces the need for those patients to raise funds to purchase illicit drugs on the black market, thus providing them time to resume employment, conventional relationships, and connections with others. These forces combine to facilitate their recovery.

Methadone and buprenorphine are common medications for opioid use disorder (MOUD). They are a form of opioid-replacement therapy that involves replacing a usually illegal opioid such as heroin (diacetylmorphine or diamorphine) or illicit fentanyl with a legal one that is less sedative and euphoric. The purpose of opioid-replacement therapy is to help avoid withdrawal, reduce drug cravings, and eliminate the euphoria associated with nonmedical drug use. Clinicians who treat addiction aim to facilitate a resumption of stability in the user's life, end the spread of disease through needle sharing, reduce the risk of overdose, and, over time, wean the user off the replacement drug. Some people with OUD stay on a MOUD indefinitely.

The DEA classifies methadone as a Schedule II drug (medically useful with a high potential for abuse). Clinicians have used methadone as a MOUD for years in the United States and many other developed countries. Twenty milligrams of oral methadone has roughly the same potency as 5 milligrams of intravenous heroin, which is approximately 2.5 times the strength of intravenous morphine.[47]

Buprenorphine is another drug that clinicians use to treat pain or OUD. Patients usually take buprenorphine and methadone orally. Buprenorphine is a partial opioid agonist, meaning that it partially activates opioid receptors. It can sometimes precipitate withdrawal in patients with opioid dependency, so to avoid this practitioners will usually prescribe buprenorphine to patients after an opioid-free interval.

Methadone is a full agonist, meaning it fully activates receptor sites. Because patients can take the drug in amounts that occupy all the opioid receptors, it is more effective in treating patients who have grown dependent on high doses of opioids. Because buprenorphine is only a partial agonist, it causes less respiratory depression than methadone and thus has less overdose potential.

Clinicians treating addiction have used methadone for a long time, but they have used buprenorphine for a shorter period, so few good studies compare the two to determine the better treatment. A 2003 Cochrane review found buprenorphine to be considerably less successful than methadone in retaining patients in treatment.[48] A 2015 study by Adam Peddicord and others concluded that "the research does not indicate that one medication is a better option than the other. This decision must be based on an individual basis after reviewing important patient factors such as health status and access to the medication."[49] A May 2023 systematic review by Australian researchers Louisa Degenhardt and colleagues found no statistically significant differences in mortality between methadone and sublingual buprenorphine, even though more patients dropped out of the buprenorphine arm.[50]

A different approach to medication-assisted therapy uses naltrexone, which is sold under the brand name Vivitrol. Naltrexone is a long-acting opioid antagonist that blocks opioid receptors, similar to the overdose antidote naloxone. Thus, it may precipitate withdrawal symptoms in patients physically dependent on opioids. It can be taken orally, with the effects lasting 24 to 48 hours, or injected intramuscularly in an extended-release form every month. For it to be effective, treatment should start only after the patient has detoxified. A 2011 analysis showed that oral naltrexone therapy had high dropout rates because of its short duration of action and was no better than a placebo, with or without corresponding psychotherapy.[51]

In 2020, Sarah Wakeman and others published comparative effectiveness research on more than 40,000 adults with OUD using six different therapeutic pathways: inpatient detoxification or residential services, intensive behavioral health, nonintensive behavioral health, buprenorphine or methadone, naltrexone, or no treatment. Their study found that compared to the other treatments, methadone and buprenorphine were the only treatments associated with reduced overdoses and hospitalizations for acute opioid-related illnesses.[52]

Finally, another MOUD is diacetylmorphine—heroin. Heroin maintenance treatment began in Switzerland in 1994 for people with OUD who failed methadone treatment. Since then, programs have started in Spain (2003), Canada (2005), Germany (2009), the Netherlands (2009), and the United Kingdom (2019). A 2011 analysis comparing heroin maintenance treatment to other MOUDs concluded that it is an effective adjunct in treating OUD, particularly in patients for whom methadone treatment was unsuccessful.[53]

The Drug Addiction Treatment Act of 2000 placed numerous restrictions on clinicians wishing to prescribe buprenorphine for OUD, initially allowing only physicians to prescribe the drug and limiting the number of patients that clinicians may treat.[54] In December 2022, Congress passed legislation removing many of the more onerous restrictions and permitting some nonphysician clinicians (e.g., nurse practitioners) to prescribe buprenorphine for OUD in primary care settings. Prescribers must still follow regulations from the DEA and the Substance Abuse and Mental Health Services Administration.[55] Few new clinicians have begun treating OUD with buprenorphine since the reform took effect.[56] One reason for this is that law enforcement surveils clinicians who treat OUD, and clinicians fear this might make them susceptible to high-profile police raids that could destroy their careers.[57]

The government only lets clinicians prescribe methadone to treat pain. In the United States, before 1972 primary care physicians would prescribe methadone to people with OUD.[58] Since 1972, however, only government-approved opioid treatment programs (OTPs) have been able to dispense methadone to treat OUD. The Comprehensive Drug Abuse Prevention and Control Act of 1970 required the secretary of the

Department of Health and Human Services to "determine the appropriate methods of professional practice in the medical treatment of the narcotic addiction of various classes of narcotics addicts."[59] As a result, the Substance Abuse and Mental Health Services Administration imposes regulations and restrictions on organizations that seek to operate OTPs. These programs must obtain certification from the DEA to operate a narcotics treatment program. States must also license OTPs, thus imposing additional regulations and restrictions on them.

The various layers of regulations obstruct the proliferation of OTPs and impede access to methadone treatment by placing burdensome requirements on patients who seek it. Federal and state regulations discriminate against, stigmatize, and dehumanize opioid users. Government obstacles explain why only about 400,000 people with OUD received methadone in 2019, although 1.6 million US residents reported that they developed OUD that year.[60]

In Canada, Australia, and the United Kingdom, clinicians have been using methadone to treat OUD in primary care settings and have prescribed take-home methadone since the late 1960s. They may exercise their medical judgment in deciding the timing and amount of take-home methadone.[61]

Clinicians and patients in the United States deserve the same freedom. American lawmakers should enable patients with OUD to receive methadone treatment from sources other than government-approved OTPs. Providers should include office-based addiction specialists, primary care physicians, nurse practitioners, and physician assistants. These treatment options can coexist with more traditional inpatient and outpatient treatment programs.[62]

Treating substance use disorder is complicated. Practitioners must commit to developing close relationships with their patients, taking the time for deep discussions, and monitoring them closely. Not every primary care practitioner will feel competent to treat patients with

OUD and will refer those patients to appropriate practitioners. However, allowing all primary care providers to provide methadone treatment would significantly expand treatment options and access to care.

If enabling people with OUD to access methadone treatment through primary care clinicians is not politically feasible, then lawmakers should allow patients to obtain methadone treatment from addiction medicine specialists in an office setting. Lawmakers should avoid enacting timelines, dosages, and amounts of take-home methadone that clinicians may prescribe. They should defer to clinicians' expertise and judgment.

As of the summer of 2024, Congress is considering the Modernizing Opioid Treatment Access Act, which would allow board-certified addiction specialists to treat people with OUD in their offices using methadone. If Congress enacts the bill and the president signs it into law, it will be a small step in the right direction—a small step because there are not nearly enough board-certified addiction specialists to serve patients who are seeking methadone treatment for OUD, assuming they are all taking new patients.[63]

Voluntary Treatment Yes, Coerced Treatment No

Lawmakers in several states, notably including the most populous state, California, are proposing laws aimed at coercing people whom police arrest and courts convict for possessing illicit drugs to enter drug rehabilitation programs or face jail time.[64] Oregon became the most recent state to embrace coercive treatment when lawmakers there throttled the state's short-lived experiment with drug decriminalization in March 2024.[65] According to the Northeastern University Center for Health Policy and Law, 38 states currently authorize judges to commit people to addiction treatment facilities. The median duration of commitment is 90 days. Sixteen states force people to undergo treatment for substance use disorder without their consent.[66]

One problem with this policy is that many people who are convicted of illegal drug possession are not addicted to the drug and do not need treatment. Research shows that 80 to 90 percent of adults who indulge in illicit drug use don't become addicted.[67] But there are other problems with courts ordering people who use drugs to undergo treatment.

All drug rehab programs are not the same. Prosecutors and judges should not be deciding what method of treatment to employ on a patient. Many courts are partial to sending convicts to 12-step abstinence-only programs, despite evidence showing that these programs have a high failure rate.[68]

There is a lot of truth to the old joke that starts with the question: "How many psychiatrists does it take to change a light bulb?" Answer: "Only one—but it must really want to change." Mental health professionals know that if their patients are not deeply motivated, they are unlikely to be successful in treating their mental health disorders.

Addiction is a compulsive behavioral disorder characterized by continually using a substance or engaging in an activity despite the negative consequences. Jail is a negative consequence. Neither jail nor the less negative alternative of a forced stay in a rehab facility are likely to make anyone overcome their addiction unless they are deeply motivated to do so at the outset. Research shows that involuntary treatment usually doesn't work.[69] In fact, research suggests that coercing drug treatment might increase the risk of subsequent overdose.[70] A 2016 systematic review of research on compulsory rehab found no evidence of improved outcomes, with some studies suggesting that compulsory rehab did more harm than good.[71] A 2017 report by the Massachusetts Department of Public Health found that fatal overdoses were twice as high among people who were subjected to compulsory treatment compared to those who entered treatment voluntarily.[72] This is because patients complete mandatory treatment but still retain their underlying compulsive disorder. After release from the treatment program, they have a high relapse rate.[73] Because they had abstained from drug use while in treatment, their tolerance level has dropped, and they are more prone to overdose when they resume taking their usual dose of the drug.

To be sure, there are some examples of people who respond well to compulsory treatment, but such patients are highly motivated when treatment begins. People who might fit that description include commercial airline pilots or medical doctors, who face losing their license—and their careers—unless they enter drug rehab. But they are exceptions to the rule.

However, the most important reason why coercive treatment is wrong is that it is an affront to personal autonomy. Treatment versus jail time does not equal informed consent.

Safer Supply

In 2020, the Canadian Province of British Columbia became the first jurisdiction to permit clinicians to prescribe hydromorphone (Dilaudid) to OUD patients to get them to switch from dangerous street drugs to safer pharmaceutical-grade prescription pain pills. Hydromorphone is roughly twice the potency of diacetylmorphine (heroin).[74] British Columbia makes taxpayers foot the bill when these patients fill prescriptions at pharmacies. The government should not force British Columbia residents to pay for other people's prescriptions.

The "safer supply" rationale is based on experiences earlier this century with the so-called prescription pain pill crisis. In chapter 6 I explained how nonmedical drug users migrated first to heroin and then to fentanyl when the supply of diverted prescription pain pills dried up. The overdose rate began climbing as they migrated to harder street drugs. To this day, many nonmedical users seek prescription pain pills on the black market, often only to succumb to a fentanyl overdose from counterfeit pain pills.[75] Had the supply of pharmaceutical-grade prescription pain pills remained constant, the overdose rate might not have skyrocketed. The safer supply policy tacitly acknowledges that government crackdowns on clinicians prescribing pain pills exacerbated the overdose crisis.

Researchers are still collecting and analyzing data to assess the impact of safer supply. Currently, there is not enough data to draw any conclusions.[76]

The Optimal Harm-Reduction Strategy

If the government ended its war on drugs, people would be able to purchase them from legal suppliers. They would comparison shop. They would know with confidence the drugs they were buying, the dosage, and the purity. Drug makers would compete on price and quality. The market, the civil tort system, and the criminal justice system would hold drug makers accountable for any harm they inflict on consumers.

As with currently legal drugs, such as alcohol and tobacco, people would be wise to employ harm-reduction strategies when consuming them. But the harm-reduction strategy that would yield the most bang for the buck is to end drug prohibition.

CHAPTER 12

The Schloendorff Legacy

I introduced this book by recounting the story of Mary Schloendorff and her fight for patient autonomy, culminating in the 1914 New York Appeals Court case *Schloendorff v. Society of New York Hospital*. That pivotal moment planted the seeds for the development of the 20th-century concept of patient autonomy within the medical community. As we entered the 21st century, health care professionals embraced and championed autonomy in all aspects of medicine. Health care professionals are committed to treating patients only if they have informed consent and respect their refusal. Today, as a profession, medical doctors take patient autonomy as seriously as libertarians do.

Regrettably, as this book has demonstrated, the doctor-patient relationship now involves more than the doctor and the patient. Government, at both the national and local level, has stepped in, usually with good intentions, in ways that ignore or violate patient autonomy. This book catalogs several ways that government does this and suggests ways for lawmakers and policymakers to rectify those transgressions.

Medical students have been reciting versions of the Hippocratic oath at graduation ceremonies for centuries. Over the past 27 years, many schools began conducting "white coat ceremonies" for entering medical students, where they recite these oaths. In recent years, schools have allowed faculty or students to compose oaths that significantly depart from tradition. None of the currently used oaths, dating back to the original Oath of Hippocrates of Kos, prioritize or consistently apply a commitment to individual patient autonomy or respect patients' rights to self-medicate and to seek treatment from any health care provider they choose.

The oath of Hippocrates dates to the 5th century BCE. Medical schools worldwide have been administering modern versions of the oath to graduating students, and medical schools in the United States are no exception.[1] Over time, many medical schools have created their own unique version of the oath.

In 1948, the World Medical Association drafted a version of the Hippocratic oath called the Declaration of Geneva.[2] It published updated versions in 1968, 1983, 1994, 2005, and 2006. In 1964, Louis Lasagna, the academic dean of Tufts University School of Medicine, drafted a modern version of the Hippocratic oath that many United States medical schools used for the next four decades.[3]

In 1993, Columbia University College of Physicians and Surgeons became the first medical school to hold a white coat ceremony for students beginning their medical education. Students, donning the physician's white coat for the first time, took the oath during this welcoming ceremony instead of at graduation.[4] Many other medical schools later adopted this ritual.

A 2015 survey of 111 medical schools in the United States and Canada found that 80 had students recite oaths at graduation and 72 had white-coat oaths.[5] The survey found that more than half of the schools no longer hewed to the Lasagna or Geneva versions of the oath that had been popular since the end of World War II. Many medical schools drafted their unique versions of the oath, sometimes written by faculty committees. Frequently, student class representatives composed the oaths. For example, the University of Pittsburgh School of Medicine created its version of the oath in 1883 and updated it for the first time in 2020.[6]

The newer versions stray significantly from the long-established oaths. They still retain a few elements of the more traditional oaths, notably pledges to respect patient privacy, avoid harm, and defend the profession's uprightness. Most oaths still commit to sharing and advancing knowledge and preventing and treating disease.[7] Yet no oath, including the oath of Hippocrates, makes more than a passing mention of respecting patients' rights as sovereign autonomous adults.

The Hippocratic Oath

The following is the 5th century BCE Oath of Hippocrates of Kos, translated from ancient Greek:

> I swear by Apollo the physician, by Aesculapius, Hygeia, and Panacea, and I take to witness all the gods, all the goddesses, to keep according to my ability and judgment the following oath:
>
> To consider dear to me as my parents him who taught me this art; to live in common with him and if necessary to share my goods with him; to look upon his children as my own brothers, to teach them this art if they so desire without fee or written promise; to impart to my sons and the sons of the master who taught me and to the disciples who have enrolled themselves and have agreed to the rules of the profession, but to these alone, the precepts and the instruction. I will prescribe regimen for the good of my patients according to my ability and my judgment and never do harm to anyone. To please no one will I prescribe a deadly drug, nor give advice which may cause his death. Nor will I give a woman a pessary to procure abortion. But I will preserve the purity of my life and my art. I will not cut for stone, even for patients in whom the disease is manifest; I will leave this operation to be performed by specialists in this art. In every house where I come I will enter only for the good of my patients,

keeping myself far from all intentional ill-doing and all seduction, and especially from the pleasures of love with women or with men, be they free or slaves. All that may come to my knowledge in the exercise of my profession or outside of my profession or in daily commerce with men, which ought not to be spread abroad, I will keep secret and never reveal. If I keep this oath faithfully, may I enjoy my life and practice my art, respected by all men and in all times; but if I swerve from it or violate it, may the reverse be my lot.[8]

Lasagna Version of Hippocratic Oath

In 1964, Tufts University School of Medicine academic dean Louis Lasagna wrote this version of the Hippocratic oath, which students, including me, in many American medical schools, recited for much of the late 20th century:

I swear to fulfill, to the best of my ability and judgment, this covenant:

I will respect the hard-won scientific gains of those physicians in whose steps I walk, and gladly share such knowledge as is mine with those who are to follow;

I will apply, for the benefit of the sick, all measures which are required, avoiding those twin traps of overtreatment and therapeutic nihilism.

I will remember that there is art to medicine as well as science, and that warmth, sympathy and understanding may outweigh the surgeon's knife or the chemist's drug.

I will not be ashamed to say "I know not," nor will I fail to call in my colleagues when the skills of another are needed for a patient's recovery.

I will respect the privacy of my patients, for their problems are not disclosed to me that the world may know. Most especially must I tread with care in matters of life and death. If it is given me to save a life, all thanks. But it may also be within my power to take a life;

this awesome responsibility must be faced with great humbleness and awareness of my own frailty. Above all, I must not play at God.

I will remember that I do not treat a fever chart, a cancerous growth, but a sick human being, whose illness may affect the person's family and economic stability. My responsibility includes these related problems, if I am to care adequately for the sick.

I will prevent disease whenever I can, for prevention is preferable to cure.

I will remember that I remain a member of society, with special obligations to all my fellow human beings, those sound of mind and body, as well as the infirm.

If I do not violate this oath, may I enjoy life and art, respected while I live and remembered with affection hereafter. May I always act so as to preserve the finest traditions of my calling and may I long experience the joy of healing those who seek my help.[9]

A Hippocratic Oath for a Free Society

I propose that medical school administrators who are willing to depart from tradition adopt the following oath that prioritizes the autonomy and rights of individual patients to guide the medical profession in its noble mission to roll back government interference and restore autonomy:

As a member of this class, I swear to fulfill, to the best of my ability, this covenant:

I will respect the crucial scientific advances in medicine but will always question the assumptions my profession has inherited and judge them in the light of the latest evidence. I will gladly share any knowledge I have gleaned from years of research, study, and clinical experience with health professionals in all disciplines. I will respect my patients' autonomy, thoroughly explain all the diagnostic possibilities and therapeutic options as I understand them, offer them my best opinion and advice from among these options, and accept their decisions.

I will never examine a patient or perform a diagnostic test or procedure without informed consent. I will not be afraid to say "I don't know," and I will not hesitate to ask my colleagues for assistance or advice when I need it to care for my patient.

Even if they act against my advice and I disapprove of their choices, I will respect the right of my patients as autonomous adults to self-medicate and oppose any laws and regulations that force them to seek my permission—or permission from any other health professional, through a prescription or otherwise—to consume medications or treatments according to their independent judgment. I will respect the privacy of my patients, for when they disclose their problems to me, they expect and deserve confidentiality.

Respecting individual autonomy, I will oppose laws that punish people for choosing to consume substances or engage in activities that might potentially harm them but do not infringe on the rights of others. If patients engage in lifestyle choices or use substances against my advice that I disapprove of and deem harmful, I will offer them advice, medication, equipment, and techniques to reduce the harm that may come from their choices. I will not morally judge patients with substance use disorder, addiction, or other behavioral health problems, but I will treat them with dignity and compassion.

I will oppose all efforts, and existing laws and regulations, including professional licensing and "scope of practice" laws, that limit patients' freedom to choose a health plan or health care arrangement or prevent patients from seeking advice or care from non-physician health professionals, regardless of the type of health care service such professionals offer and irrespective of their level of expertise and training.

I will remember that there is an art to medicine as well as a science and that warmth, sympathy, and understanding are crucial to the healing process. I will remember that treating pain is crucial to my professional mission to ease human suffering. I will use my best judgment and follow my conscience to prescribe adequate treatments for my patients who are in pain, despite the prejudices of public policymakers and law enforcement who might try to interfere.

I will remember that I do not treat a medical chart, a set of vital signs, or a cancerous growth, but a sick person whose illness may affect the person's family and economic stability. My responsibility includes helping my patient to weigh the tradeoffs, making a personal risk/benefit analysis when deciding on a therapeutic course of action, and respecting my patient's ultimate decision. I will strive to prevent disease, for prevention is preferable to cure.

I hope my patients and colleagues will remember me with respect and affection if I stay true to this oath.[10]

As fiduciaries of Mary Schloendorff's legacy, medical professionals should take the lead in the battle to roll back government intervention and restore patient autonomy.

List of Agencies, Terms, and Acronyms

advanced practice registered nurse (APRN)

Alaska Native Tribal Health Consortium (ANTHC)

American Academy of Physician Assistants (AAPA)

American Board of Family Medicine (ABFM)

American Board of Obstetrics and Gynecology (ABOG)

American Board of Pediatrics (ABP)

American Board of Surgery (ABS)

American Cancer Society Cancer Action Network (ACS CAN)

American Civil Liberties Union (ACLU)

American College of Neuropsychopharmacology (ACNP)

American College of Obstetrics and Gynecology (ACOG)

American Dental Association (ADA)

American Hospital Association (AHA)

American Hospital Formulary Service-Drug Information (AHFS-DI)

American Medical Association (AMA)

American Medical Association Drug Evaluations (AMADE)

AMA House of Delegates (AMA-HOD)

American Psychiatric Association (APA)

American Public Health Association (APHA)

American Society of Addiction Medicine (ASAM)

ambulatory surgery center (ASC)

attention-deficit/hyperactivity disorder (ADHD)

assistant physicians (AP)

bachelor of oral health (BOH)

behind the counter (BTC)

Centers for Medicare and Medicaid Services (CMS)

Centers for Disease Control and Prevention (CDC)

certificate of need (CON)

certified nurse midwife (CNM)

certified registered nurse anesthetist (CRNA)

clinical nurse specialist (CNS)

Combat Methamphetamine Epidemic Act (CMEA)

Commission on Dental Accreditation (CODA)

conformity européenne/European conformity (CE)

Council on Medical Education (CME)

Council on Pharmacy and Chemistry (CPC)

Department of Defense (DOD)

department of public health (DPH)

dimethyltryptamine (DMT)

direct-to-consumer (DTC)

doctor of pharmacology (PharmD)

Drug Enforcement Administration (DEA)

Duchenne muscular dystrophy (DMD)

Educational Commission for Foreign Medical Graduates (ECFMG)

exchange visitor (EV)

Federal Aviation Administration (FAA)

Federal Bureau of Narcotics (FBN)

Federal Trade Commission (FTC)

Food and Drug Administration (FDA)

Food, Drug, and Cosmetic Act (FDCA)

Government Accountability Office (GAO)

Health and Human Services (HHS)

health professional shortage area (HPSA)

Health Resources and Services Administration (HRSA)

Indian Health Service (IHS)

International Classification of Diseases, 11th Revision (ICD 11)

international medical graduate (IMG)

internet addiction disorder (IAD)

Liaison Committee on Medical Education (LCME)

lysergic acid diethylamide (LSD)

medication for opioid use disorder (MOUD)

methylenedioxymethamphetamine (MDMA) (ecstasy)

Middle East respiratory syndrome (MERS)

National Academies of Sciences, Engineering, and Medicine (NASEM)

National Board of Medical Examiners (NBME)

National Commission on Certification of Physician Assistants (NCCPA)

National Comprehensive Cancer Network (NCCN)

National Council for Mental Wellbeing (no official acronym)

National Institute on Drug Abuse (NIDA)

National Institute of Mental Health (NIMH)

National Medical Association (NMA)

National Resident Matching Program (NRMP)

National Student Internship Committee (NSIC)

National Survey on Drug Use and Health (NSDUH)

nicotine replacement therapy (NRT)

neutral protamine Hagedorn insulin (NPH insulin)

nurse practitioner (NP)

obstetrician-gynecologist (ob-gyn)

opioid use disorder (OUD)

opioid treatment programs (OTP)

overdose prevention center (OPC)

over the counter (OTC)

phenyl-2-propanone (P2P)

physician assistant (PA)

post-exposure prophylaxis (PEP)

post-traumatic stress disorder (PTSD)

pre-exposure prophylaxis (PrEP)

prescribing psychologist (RxP)

Psychopharmacology Exam for Psychologists (PEP)

registered nurse (RN)

Substance Abuse and Mental Health Services Administration
   (SAMHSA)

Supplemental Offer and Acceptance Program (SOAP)

syringe services program (SSP)

tetrahydrocannabinol (THC)

United States Bureau of Chemistry; Food, Drug, and Insecticide
    Administration (see Food and Drug Administration [FDA])
United States Congressional Joint Economic Committee (JEC)
United States Public Health Service Commissioned Corps (USPHSCC)
United States Pharmacopeia/United States Pharmacopeial
    Convention (USP)
United States Pharmacopeia and National Formulary (USP-NF)
United States Pharmacopeia Drug Information (USP-DI)

Veterans Health Administration (VHA)

World Health Organization (WHO)
World Medical Association (WMA)

ACKNOWLEDGMENTS

I want to thank Michael Cannon, Cato's director of health policy studies, for inspiring me to write this book, offering invaluable suggestions, even suggesting its title, and for helping me view public policy in general and health policy in particular through a lens that presumes liberty and autonomy. Thanks must also go to Alex Nowrasteh, Cato's vice president for economic and social policy studies, for his encouragement and support. This book would not have been possible without my outstanding editors, Eleanor O'Connor and Ivan Osorio, whose invaluable recommendations guided me through the writing process. As a former policy analyst, Ivan provided constructive criticisms that strengthened my arguments. I am indebted to Karen Garvin for her meticulous copyediting. I also thank Alex Kolonchin for his editorial assistance. I am grateful to Dr. Ross Levatter for his helpful feedback and suggestions, especially regarding chapter 12. Finally, I want to thank my wife, Meg. As an English literature major with no background in the health sciences, she diligently scanned my text, pointing out language that was too jargony for a general audience—when she wasn't patiently enduring my hours in seclusion as I wrote this book.

NOTES

Introduction

1. Lydia A. Bazzano, Jaquail Durant, and Paula Rhode Brantley, "A Modern History of Informed Consent and the Role of Key Information," *Ochsner Journal* 21, no. 1 (2021): 81–85.
2. Emphasis added. *Schloendorff v. New York Hospital*, 211 N.Y. 125 (N.Y. 1914), Casetext. The court determined that Schloendorff's doctors had committed an assault. It nevertheless ruled against her because she had sued the hospital, which the court found not liable for the actions of the doctors who practiced there.
3. Daniel K. Sokol, "How the Doctor's Nose Has Shortened over Time; a Historical Overview of the Truth-Telling Debate in the Doctor-Patient Relationship," *Journal of the Royal Society of Medicine* 99, no. 12 (December 2006): 632–36.
4. Sokol, "How the Doctor's Nose Has Shortened over Time."

Chapter 1

1. John Christman, "Autonomy in Moral and Political Philosophy," *Stanford Encyclopedia of Philosophy*, ed. Edward N. Zalta (Fall 2020 edition).
2. Tom L. Beauchamp and James F. Childress, *Principles of Biomedical Ethics*, 4th ed. (New York: Oxford University Press, 1994).
3. Lydia A. Bazzano, Jaquail Durant, and Paula Rhode Brantley, "A Modern History of Informed Consent and the Role of Key Information," *Ochsner Journal* 21, no. 1 (March 2021): 81–85.
4. Karl O. Nakken and Antonia Villagran, "From Hystero Epilepsy to Nonepileptic Seizure," *Tidsskr Nor Legeforen* 141 (2021). In the 19th and early 20th century many physicians believed that seizures and hysteria in women were caused by a "wandering" uterus. The word "hysteria" derives from the Greek word for womb, *hystera*.
5. Bazzano, Durant, and Brantley, "A Modern History of Informed Consent and the Role of Key Information."
6. *Mohr v. Williams*, 95 Minn. 261, 104 N.W. 12.
7. Lydia A. Bazzano, Jaquail Durant, and Paula Rhode Brantley, "A Modern History of Informed Consent and the Role of Key Information," *Ochsner Journal* 21 (Spring 2021): 81–85.
8. *Schloendorff v. Society of New York Hosp.*, 105 N.E. 92, 93 (N.Y. 1914).
9. *Canterbury v. Spence*, 464 F.2d 772 (D.C. Cir. 1972).
10. David William Archard, "Children's Rights," *Stanford Encyclopedia of Philosophy*, ed. Edward N. Zalta and Uri Nodelman, (Spring 2023 edition).
11. Eugene Volokh, "Liberty and Parental Rights," *The Volokh Conspiracy* (blog), June 15, 2011.
12. Jeffrey A. Singer, "Let Intersex Individuals Choose Their Destiny," *Orange County Register*, July 24, 2019; and Ganny Belloni, "Transgender Youth Care Targeted in Culture Battle Sweeping US," Bloomberg Law, February 21, 2023.

13. John Stuart Mill, *On Liberty and Other Essays,* ed. John Gray (New York: Oxford University Press, 2008), pp. 83–104, 117.

14. Jessica Flanigan, *Pharmaceutical Freedom: Why Patients Have a Right to Self-Medicate* (New York: Oxford University Press, 2017), p. 65n9, citing Thomas Jefferson, *Notes on the State of Virginia,* ed. Frank Shuffelton (New York, Penguin Classics, 1998), Query XVII.

15. Flanigan, *Pharmaceutical Freedom,* p. 3.

16. Overuse and misuse of antibiotics can contribute to the development of resistant strains of bacteria, rendering existing antibiotics less effective in the treatment of infectious and communicable diseases. "High Levels of Antibiotic Resistance Found Worldwide, New Data Shows," World Health Organization (WHO), January 29, 2018; "Stop Using Antibiotics in Healthy Animals to Prevent the Spread of Antibiotic Resistance," WHO, November 7, 2017; and "WHO Updates Essential Medicines List with New Advice on Use of Antibiotics, and Adds Medicines for Hepatitis C, HIV, Tuberculosis and Cancer," WHO, June 6, 2017.

17. Stephen Eldridge, "Negative Externality," *Encyclopedia Britannica,* March 15, 2024.

18. Flanigan, *Pharmaceutical Freedom,* pp. 41–43, 88.

Chapter 2

1. Ilya Shapiro, "State Police Powers and the Constitution," Pandemics and Policy, Cato Institute, September 15, 2020; and Randy E. Barnett, "The Proper Scope of the Police Power," *Notre Dame Law Review* 79, no. 2, article 1 (2004): 429–95.

2. "State Specific Requirements for Initial Medical Licensure," Federation of State Medical Boards.

3. Brendan Murphy, "Licensing and Board Certification: What Residents Need to Know," American Medical Association, May 22, 2019.

4. Paul Starr, *The Social Transformation of American Medicine: The Rise of a Sovereign Profession and the Making of a Vast Industry* (New York: Basic Books, 1982), pp. 40–59.

5. Ronald Hamowy, "The Early Development of Medical Licensing Laws in the United States, 1875–1900," *Journal of Libertarian Studies* 3, no. 1 (1979): 75.

6. "AAMC History," Association of American Medical Colleges.

7. Robert B. Baker, "The American Medical Association and Race," *AMA Journal of Ethics* 16, no. 6 (June 2014): 479–88; Paul Starr, *The Social Transformation of American Medicine: The Rise of a Sovereign Profession and the Making of a Vast Industry,* 2nd ed. (New York: Basic Books, 2017); Hamowy, "The Early Development of Medical Licensing Laws"; Elizabeth Hlavinka, "Racial Bias in Flexner Report Permeates Medical Education Today," *MedPage Today,* June 18, 2020; Starr, *The Social Transformation of American Medicine* (1982); and Jeffrey A. Singer, "Race and Medical Licensing Laws," *Cato at Liberty* (blog), Cato Institute, June 29, 2020.

8. Baker, "The American Medical Association and Race."

9. Paul Starr, *The Social Transformation of American Medicine* (1982), p. 124.

10. Starr, *The Social Transformation of American Medicine* (1982), p. 124.

11. Jeffrey A. Singer and Richard P. Menger, "The Coronavirus Pandemic Shows the Folly of Medical Licensing Laws," *National Review*, May 29, 2020; "COVID-19 Emergency Declaration Blanket Waivers for Health Care Providers," Centers for Medicare and Medicaid Services, March 30, 2020; for state order, see, for example, "South Carolina Medical and Nursing Boards to Issue Emergency Licenses," Office of South Carolina Governor Henry McMaster, news release, March 14, 2020; "Governor Changes Licensing Laws to Fight COVID-19," KWTX 10, March 15, 2020; and Arizona HB 2569.

12. See "Section 3: Annotation," in Christina Sandefur, Byron Schlomach, and Murray Feldstein, "A Win-Win for Consumers and Professionals Alike: An Alternative to Occupational Licensing," Goldwater Institute, November 15, 2018, p. 5; "Naturopathic Licensing Status in Michigan," Michigan Association of Naturopathic Doctors; and Edward Timmons and Jarrett Skorup, "State Licensing Should only Be a Last Resort," *Detroit News*, June 2, 2018.

13. "The Complexities of Physician Supply and Demand: Projections From 2021 to 2036," prepared for the Association of American Medical Colleges by GlobalData Plc., March 2024.

14. Xiaoming Zhang et al., "Physician Workforce in the United States of America: Forecasting Nationwide Shortages," *Human Resources for Health* 18, no. 8 (February 6, 2020).

15. Elaine K. Howley, "The U.S. Physician Shortage Is Only Going to Get Worse. Here Are Potential Solutions," *Time*, July 25, 2022.

16. Emily P. Terlizzi and Jeannine S. Schiller, "Mental Health Treatment among Adults Aged 18–44: United States, 2019–2021," National Center for Health Statistics Data Brief no. 444, Centers for Disease Control and Prevention, September 2022.

17. "Mental Health Care Health Professional Shortage Areas (HPSAs)," State Health Facts, Kaiser Family Foundation, September 30, 2021, last modified April 1, 2024.

18. Clinical Nurse Specialist," Top Nursing; and Daniel Bal, "How to Become an APRN," *NurseJournal*, updated January 10, 2023.

19. Theresa Granger, "Nurse Practitioners: A Look Back and Moving Forward," USC Suzanne Dworak-Peck School of Social Work, November 10, 2017.

20. "Protect Access to Physician-Led Care," American Medical Association, 2023.

21. "Quality of Nurse Practitioner Practice," American Association of Nurse Practitioners.

22. Chuan-Fen Liu et al., "Outcomes of Primary Care Delivery by Nurse Practitioners: Utilization, Cost, and Quality of Care," *Health Services Research* 55, no. 2 (April 2020): 178–89, January 13, 2020; Anthony D. Harris et al., "The Use and Interpretation of Quasi-Experimental Studies in Medical Informatics," *Journal of the American Medical Informatics Association* 13, no. 1 (January–February 2006): 16–23. The pseudo-random element of the study addresses the confounding variable of sampling bias. The integrated model of the VHA removed the exogenous variables of patient preference and complexity of health status at the time of reassignment. In addition, the study's

large sample size accomplishes a degree of generalizability that other studies have not. This minimizes the effect of independent variables seen in other studies, thus enabling researchers to better estimate the association between NP-assigned and physician-assigned patient outcomes.

23. Liu et al., "Outcomes of Primary Care Delivery by Nurse Practitioners"; and Harris et al., "The Use and Interpretation of Quasi-Experimental Studies in Medical Informatics."

24. "NP Fact Sheet," American Association of Nurse Practitioners.

25. Ann Feeney, "Nurse Practitioner Practice Authority: A State-by-State Guide," *NurseJournal,* updated May 23, 2024.

26. "Nurse Anesthesia: How It All Started," Texas Wesleyan University, January 22, 2016.

27. Rebecca Munday, "CRNA Supervision Requirements by State," *NurseJournal,* updated November 16, 2023.

28. Brian Dulisse and Jerry Cromwell, "No Harm Found When Nurse Anesthetists Work Without Supervision by Physicians," *Health Affairs* (Project Hope) 29, no. 8 (2010): 1469–75.

29. Dulisse and Cromwell, "No Harm Found."

30. "Nurse Anesthesia: How It All Started," Texas Wesleyan University; and "CRNA Supervision Requirements by State," *NurseJournal.*

31. "About NCCPA—Our History," National Commission on Certification of Physician Assistants.

32. Thomas A. Hemphill and Gerald Knesek, "The Non-Physician Remedy to the Physician Shortage," *Regulation* 38, no. 2 (Summer 2015): 2–3.

33. "In What States Can Physician Assistants Practice Independently?," Barton Associates, June 8, 2023.

34. "Practicing Medicine in the U.S. as an International Medical Graduate," American Medical Association.

35. "History of ECFMG," Educational Commission for Foreign Medical Graduates.

36. "Practicing Medicine in the U.S. as an International Medical Graduate," American Medical Association; "History of ECFMG," Educational Commission for Foreign Medical Graduates; and Kevin Dayaratna, Paul J. Larkin Jr., and John O'Shea, "Reforming American Medical Licensure," *Harvard Journal of Law & Public Policy* 42, no. 1 (2019): 253–78.

37. David J. Bier, "Employment-Based Green Card Backlog Hits 1.2 Million in 2020," *Cato at Liberty* (blog), Cato Institute, November 20, 2020.

38. Jonathan Wolfson, "How Tennessee Is Creating New Opportunities for Doctors Trained Outside the U.S.," STAT, May 18, 2023; and S.B. 1451, "An Act to Amend Tennessee Code Annotated Title 63 Relative to Health Care," 2023 Sess. (Tenn. 2023).

39. Jeffrey A. Singer, "More States Move to Let Experienced Foreign Doctors Serve Their Patients," *Cato at Liberty* (blog), Cato Institute, March 14, 2024.

40. Alvin E. Roth, "The Origins, History, and Design of the Resident Match," *JAMA* 289, no. 7 (February 19, 2003): 909–12; and "About the National Resident Matching Program," National Resident Matching Program.

41. "Intro to the Match," National Resident Matching Program.

42. "SOAP," National Resident Matching Program.

43. Brendan Murphy, "If You're Feeling Disappointed on Match Day, You Are Not Alone," Preparing for Residency, American Medical Association, April 8, 2024; and Timothy M. Smith, "What If You Don't Match? 4 Things You Should Do," Preparing for Residency, American Medical Association, March 8, 2024.

44. Robert G. Slawson, "Medical Training in the United States Prior to the Civil War," *Journal of Evidence-Based Integrative Medicine* 17, no. 1 (September 28, 2011): 11–27; and "The Physician's Apprentice," *Yale Medicine Magazine*, Yale School of Medicine, Spring 2010.

45. "Professionally Active Primary Care Physicians by Field," Kaiser Family Foundation, January 2024; "Licensee Search—Active Licensee Only," Missouri Division of Professional Registration; Jeffrey A. Singer and Spencer Pratt, "Expand Access to Primary Care: Remove Barriers to Assistant Physicians," Cato Institute Briefing Paper no. 152, April 24, 2023.

46. Singer and Pratt, "Expand Access to Primary Care: Remove Barriers to Assistant Physicians."

47. "Mental Illness," Mental Health Information, National Institute of Mental Health, last updated March 2023.

48. Erika Edwards, "After 2-Year Decline, Suicide Rates Rise Again," *NBC News*, September 30, 2022; and Sally C. Curtin, Matthew F. Garnett, and Farida B. Ahmad, "Provisional Numbers and Rates of Suicide by Month and Demographic Characteristics: United States, 2021," Vital Statistics Rapid Release Report no. 24, National Vital Statistics System, National Center for Health Statistics, Centers for Disease Control and Prevention, September 2022.

49. "About Underlying Cause of Death, 1999–2020," CDC WONDER, Centers for Disease Control and Prevention.

50. Nina Chamlou, "How to Become a Clinical Psychologist," Psychology.org, updated August 11, 2022.

51. Michelle Andrews, "Psychologists Seek Authority to Prescribe Psychotropic Medication," *Washington Post*, March 21, 2011; and Ramin Mojtabai and Mark Olfson, "National Trends in Psychotherapy by Office-Based Psychiatrists," *Archives of General Psychiatry* 65, no. 8 (August 2008): 962–70.

52. Richard Miller, "How Much Does a Psychiatrist Cost?," BetterHelp, June 24, 2022; and Kendra Bean, "How Much Does It Cost to See a Psychiatrist without Insurance?," Mira, August 23, 2022.

53. Tara F. Bishop et al., "Acceptance of Insurance by Psychiatrists and the Implications for Access to Mental Health Care," *JAMA Psychiatry* 71, no. 2 (February 2014): 176–81.

54. "Mental Health Care Health Professional Shortage Areas (HPSAs)," State Health Facts, Kaiser Family Foundation, April 1, 2024.

55. "Health Professional Shortage Areas: Mental Health, by County, 2022," Rural Health Information Hub, July 2024; and "Over One-Third of Americans Live in Areas Lacking Mental Health Professionals," USAFacts, updated July 14, 2021.

56. "DoD Prescribing Psychologists: External Analysis, Monitoring, and Evaluation of the Program and its Participants," American College of Neuropsychopharmacology, May 1998.

57. General Accounting Office, "Prescribing Psychologists: DOD Demonstration Participants Perform Well but Have Little Effect on Readiness or Costs," Health, Education, and Human Services Division, June 1999; and Jeffrey A. Singer, "Expand Access to Mental Health Care: Remove Barriers to Psychologists Prescribing Medication," Cato Institute Briefing Paper no. 142, October 27, 2022.

58. Gagandeep Singh, "Psychologists Don't Have the Medical and Science Backgrounds Needed to Prescribe Drugs," *Arizona Mirror*, February 6, 2024.

59. "DoD Prescribing Psychologists," American College of Neuropsychopharmacology, p. 5. See also Kylin Peck, Robert McGrath, and Bryan Holbrook, "Practices of Psychologists: Replication and Extension," *Professional Psychology Research and Practice* 52, no. 3 (October 2020): 195–201.

60. Agnitra Roy Choudhury and Alicia Plemmons, "Effects of Giving Psychologists Prescriptive Authority: Evidence from a Natural Experiment in the United States," *Health Policy* 134 (2023): 104846; and Jeffrey A. Singer, "New Evidence That Prescribing Psychologists Can Save Lives," *Cato at Liberty* (blog), Cato Institute, June 7, 2023.

61. The HSRA is an agency of the US Department of Health and Human Services. "States Ranked by Shortage of Dental Providers in 2023," *Becker's Dental Review*.

62. Bradley Munson and Marko Vujicic, "Projected Supply of Dentists in the United States 2020—2040," Health Policy Institute, American Dental Association, May 2021.

63. "The Story of Dental Therapy," Arizona Dental Hygiene Association.

64. Naomi Lopez, "The Reform That Can Increase Dental Access and Affordability in Arizona," Goldwater Institute, April 10, 2017.

65. Elsa Pearson Sites, "Dental Therapists: A Solution to America's Lack of Access to Dental Care," *STAT News*, February 18, 2021.

66. Allison Corr, "What Are Dental Therapists?," Pew Charitable Trusts, October 9, 2019.

67. Lopez, "The Reform That Can Increase Dental Access and Affordability in Arizona."

68. Corr, "What are Dental Therapists?"

69. David A. Nash et al., "Dental Therapists: A Global Perspective," *International Dental Journal* 58, no. 2 (April 2008): 61–70.

70. Kelsey Mo, "Gov. Doug Ducey Signs Bill Allowing 'Dental Therapists' to Practice in Arizona," *AZCentral*, May 17, 2018.

71. "Dental Therapist (DT) and Advanced Dental Therapist (ADT)," Minnesota Department of Health.

72. Jeffrey A. Singer and Joel Strom, "It's Getting Harder to See a Dentist. Here's How State Lawmakers Can Help," *Orange County Register*, June 1, 2023.

73. Vibhuti Arya et al., National Pharmacist Workforce Study 2019, American Association of Colleges of Pharmacy, January 10, 2020.

74. Alex J. Adams, Krystalyn K. Weaver, and Jennifer Athay Adams, "Revisiting the Continuum of Pharmacist Prescriptive Authority," *Journal of the American Pharmacists Association* 63, no. 5 (2023): 1508–14.

75. Jeffrey A. Singer and Courtney M. Joslin, "How States Can Promote Health Care Access and Affordability While Enhancing Patient Autonomy," R Street Policy Study no. 214, November 23, 2020.

76. American College of Obstetricians and Gynecologists, "Over-the-Counter Access to Hormonal Contraception," American College of Obstetricians and Gynecologists, Committee Opinion no. 788, October 2019; and Jeffrey A. Singer, "All Birth Control Pills, Not Just One, Should Be Over-the-Counter," *Reason*, July 14, 2023.

77. National Alliance of State Pharmacy Associations, "Pharmacist Prescribing: Statewide Protocols for Hormonal Contraceptives," National Alliance of State Pharmacy Associations; and Jeffrey A. Singer, "Arizona Governor Tries to Bring Some Arizona Women Another Step Closer to Health Care Autonomy," *Cato at Liberty* (blog), Cato Institute, July 7, 2023.

78. Laurel Wamsley, "California to Make HIV Prevention Drugs Available Without a Prescription," *NPR*, October 8, 2019; and Jeffrey A. Singer, "Add PrEP and PEP to the List of Drugs the FDA Should Make OTC," *Cato at Liberty* (blog) Cato Institute, October 11, 2019.

79. "Pharmacist Prescribing: Statewide Protocols for HIV PrEP and PEP," National Alliance of State Pharmacy Associations, December 9, 2022.

80. "Pharmacist Immunization Authority," National Alliance of State Pharmacy Associations, April 25, 2023.

81. Holly Payne, "How Do Pharmacists in Other Countries Prescribe?," *The Medical Republic*, September 27, 2022; and "Specified Prescription Medicines for Designated Pharmacist Prescribers," New Zealand Government, October 8, 2021.

82. Anita McDonald, "Opinion: Let Doctors, Pharmacists Do What They Do Best," *Edmonton Journal*, updated March 14, 2023.

83. "What Pharmacists Can Do across Canada," Canadian Pharmacists Association.

84. Dave L. Dixon, Karissa Johnston, and Julie Patterson, "Cost-Effectiveness of Pharmacist Prescribing for Managing Hypertension in the United States," *JAMA Network Open* 6, no. 11 (November 3, 2023).

85. Marc Joffe, "Idaho Leads the Nation toward Expanding Pharmacists' Scope of Practice," *Cato at Liberty* (blog), Cato Institute, August 14, 2023.

86. "New Legislation Impacting Your Profession," Florida Board of Pharmacy, June 29, 2020.

87. "2020 FMA Legislative Report," Florida Medical Association.

88. Shirley V. Svorny, "Beyond Medical Licensure," *Regulation* 38, no. 1 (Spring 2015): 26–29; Shirley V. Svorny, "Medical Licensing: An Obstacle to Affordable, Quality Care," Cato Institute Policy Analysis no. 621, September 17, 2008; and Shirley Svorny and Michael F. Cannon, "Health Care Workforce Reform: COVID-19 Spotlights Need for Changes to Clinician Licensing," Cato Institute Policy Analysis no. 899, August 4, 2020.

89. Sandefur, Schlomach, and Feldstein, "A Win-Win for Consumers and Professionals Alike."

90. Matt Shafer, "Understanding Arizona's Universal Occupational Licensing Recognition Bill," Occupational Licensure Policy, Council of State Governments, June 24, 2019; J. D. Tuccille, "Ohio to Honor Occupational

Licenses from Other States," *Reason*, January 18, 2023; Jeffrey A. Singer and Michael D. Tanner, "Arizona Leads the Way in Licensing Reform," *Arizona Capitol Times*, October 29, 2020; and "Governor DeWine Signs Bills into Law," Office of Ohio Governor Mike DeWine, January 2, 2023.

Chapter 3

1. National Health Planning and Resources Development Act, Pub. L. No. 93-641, 88 Stat. 2225 (1975).

2. "Certificate of Need State Laws," National Conference of State Legislatures, updated February 26, 2024.

3. Matthew D. Mitchell, "Do Certificate-of-Need Laws Limit Spending?," Mercatus Center at George Mason University, May 2016.

4. Matthew McGough et al., "How Has U.S. Spending on Healthcare Changed over Time?," Peterson-KFF Health System Tracker, December 15, 2023.

5. Adney Rakotoniaina and Johanna Butler, "50-State Scan of State Certificate-of-Need Programs," National Academy for State Health Policy, May 22, 2020; and "Certificate of Need State Laws," National Conference of State Legislatures, updated February 26, 2024.

6. Jennifer Thomas, "Carolinas HealthCare Asks Court to Block Fort Mill Hospital," *Charlotte Business Journal*, January 30, 2015.

7. Rebecca Hanchett, "Kentucky House Committee Nixes Certificate of Need Bill," *Link NKY*, March 21, 2024. I provided this testimony to the Kentucky legislature's Special Committee Certificate of Need Task Force on November 23, 2023: Jeffrey A. Singer, "Testimony Before the Kentucky Special Committee Certificate of Need Task Force," Cato Institute, November 20, 2023.

8. "Certificate of Need (CON) Law Series Part III: CON and the Changing Landscape of Healthcare," Health Capital Topics 5, no. 11 (November 2012): 1–2.

9. National Health Planning and Resources Development Act, Pub. L. No. 93-641, 88 Stat. 2225 (1975).

10. Claire Wallace, "The States That Do, Do Not Have CON Laws for ASCs," Becker's *ASC Review*, February 19, 2024.

11. Momotazur Rahman et al., "The Impact of Certificate-of-Need Laws on Nursing Home and Home Health Care Expenditures," *Journal of Medical Care Research and Review* 73 no. 1 (July 2015): 85–105.

12. "Choose Home Care Act," Morning Consult, Partnership for Home Quality Healthcare, polling presentation, August 2021.

13. Thomas Stratmann and Christopher Koopman, "Entry Regulation and Rural Health Care: Certificate-of-Need Laws, Ambulatory Surgery Centers, and Community Hospitals," Mercatus Center, George Mason University, February 18, 2016.

14. Thomas Stratmann and Matthew C. Baker, "Examining Certificate-of-Need Laws in the Context of the Rural Health Crisis," Mercatus Center at George Mason University, July 29, 2020.

15. Alice Proujansky, "Why Black Women Are Rejecting Hospitals in Search of Better Births," *New York Times*, March 11, 2021.

16. Erin K. George, "Birth Center Breastfeeding Rates: A Literature Review," *American Journal of Maternal/Child Nursing* 47, no. 6 (December 2022): 310–17; Jill Alliman, Kate Bauer, and Trinisha Williams, "Freestanding Birth Centers," *Journal of Perinatal Education* 31, no. 1 (January 1, 2022): 8–13; Rachel R. Hardeman et al., "Roots Community Birth Center: A Culturally-Centered Care Model for Improving Value and Equity in Childbirth," *Healthcare* 8, no. 1 (March 2020): 100367; Susan Rutledge Stapleton, Cara Osborne, and Jessica Illuzzi, "Outcomes of Care in Birth Centers: Demonstration of a Durable Model," *Journal of Midwifery & Women's Health* 58, no. 1 (January 30, 2013): 3–14.

17. "Position Statement: Certificate of Need," American Association of Birth Centers.

18. Tara Law, "Home Births Rose During the Pandemic, Study Shows," *Time*, November 17, 2022; and Nicole Harris, "Your Guide to Home Birth," *Parents*, updated September 6, 2023.

19. Shannon Najmabadi, "Your Ambulance Is on the Way. ETA: 65 Minutes," *Wall Street Journal*, November 16, 2023.

20. Yvonne Jonk et al., "Ambulance Deserts: Geographic Disparities in the Provision of Ambulance Services," Maine Rural Health Research Center, Muskie School of Public Service, University of Southern Maine, May 2023.

21. Jonk et al., "Ambulance Deserts."

22. Najmabadi, "Your Ambulance Is on the Way."

23. Jeffrey A. Singer, "Repealing Certificate of Need Laws Should Help Irrigate America's 'Ambulance Deserts,'" *Cato at Liberty* (blog), Cato Institute, November 17, 2023.

24. Angela C. Erickson, "States Are Suspending Certificate of Need Laws in the Wake of COVID-19 but the Damage Might Already Be Done," Pacific Legal Foundation, January 11, 2021; and Moriah Lawrence and Angela C. Erickson, "States That Suspended Certificate of Need Laws Saved Lives," Pacific Legal Foundation, August 19, 2020.

25. Christina Sandefur, "Competitor's Veto: State Certificate of Need Laws Violate State Prohibitions on Monopolies," Regulatory Transparency Project of the Federalist Society, February 26, 2020.

Chapter 4

1. Kate Grindlay, Bridgit Burns, and Daniel Grossman, "Prescription Requirements and Over-the-Counter Access to Oral Contraceptives: A Global Review," *Contraception* 88, no. 1 (July 2013): 91–96.

2. Kimberly Daniels and Joyce C. Abma, "Current Contraceptive Status among Women Aged 15–49: United States, 2017–2019," NCHS Data Brief no. 388 (Hyattsville, MD: National Center for Health Statistics, 2020); "Key Statistics from the National Survey of Family Growth," Centers for Disease Control and Prevention, last reviewed November 8, 2021; Kimberly Daniels, William D. Mosher, and Jo Jones, "Contraceptive Methods Women Have Ever Used: United States, 1982–2010," National Health Statistics Reports no. 62, US Centers for Disease Control and Prevention, February 14, 2013, p. 4.

3. Susannah Snider, "The Cost of Birth Control," *US News & World Report*, May 2, 2019.

4. Kate Grindlay and Daniel Grossman, "Prescription Birth Control Access among U.S. Women at Risk of Unintended Pregnancy," *Journal of Women's Health* 25, no. 3 (March 2016): 249–54.

5. Holly Mead, "Making Birth Control More Accessible to Women: A Cost-Benefit Analysis of Over-the-Counter Oral Contraceptives," Institute for Women's Policy Research, IWPR Publication no. B236, February 2001. The institute submitted this cost-benefit analysis and its recommendation to the US Food and Drug Administration in June 2000.

6. Mead, "Making Birth Control More Accessible to Women."

7. "Over-the-Counter Oral Contraceptives," American Academy of Family Physicians; and "AMA Urges FDA to Make Oral Contraceptive Available Over the Counter," American Medical Association, June 15, 2022.

8. Sarah Toy, "FDA Approves First Over-the-Counter Birth-Control Pill," *Wall Street Journal*, July 13, 2023.

9. Josh Bloom and Jeffrey A. Singer, "FDA Might Approve Over-the-Counter Sales of One Birth Control Pill. Now It's Time to Approve All the Rest," *Reason*, May 10, 2023.

10. "Progestin-Only Contraceptives," *American Family Physician* 62, no. 8 (October 2000): 1849–50.

11. "Plan B One-Step," website.

12. *Tummino v. Hamburg*, United States District Court, Eastern District of New York, No. 12-CV-763 (ERK)(VVP); Michael D. Shear and Pam Belluck, "U.S. Drops Bid to Limit Sales of Morning-After Pill," *New York Times*, June 10, 2013; and Jeffrey A. Singer and Michael F. Cannon, "Drug Reformation: End Government's Power to Require Prescriptions," Cato Institute White Paper, October 20, 2020, pp. 18–20.

13. "George Mason University in Virginia and colleges and universities in California and Pennsylvania have installed vending machines that dispense the contraceptive pill called Plan B, or a generic version that can be purchased over the counter in stores." Debbie Truong, "Women at Two Va. Universities Wanted More Access to the Morning-After Pill. So They Took 'Matters into Their Own Hands,'" *Washington Post*, May 19, 2019; and Max Blau, "The 'Uber for Birth Control' Expands in Conservative States, Opening a New Front in War over Contraception," *STAT*, October 24, 2017.

14. Susana Ronconi, "Learning from Italy's Lead on Naloxone," Voices, Open Society Foundations, March 30, 2017.

15. Eric Berger, "Narcan Price Hikes Troubling as Opioid Epidemic Rages On," *Annals of Emergency Medicine* 70, no. 4 (October 2017): 17A–19A; Singer and Cannon, "Drug Reformation," pp. 25–31.

16. Jeffrey A. Singer, "Why Doesn't the Surgeon General Seek FDA Reclassification of Naloxone to OTC?," *Cato at Liberty* (blog), Cato Institute, April 5, 2018; and Jeffrey A. Singer, "Governors' Standing Orders Can Lower Healthcare Costs," commentary, Cato Institute, February 12, 2020.

17. Julie Wernau, "Narcan Maker Gets Fast-Tracked for Over-the-Counter Nasal Spray," *Wall Street Journal*, December 6, 2022; and Jeffrey A. Singer, "Americans May Finally Get Access to OTC Naloxone," *Cato at Liberty* (blog), Cato Institute, December 7, 2022.

18. Jan Hoffman, "Over-the-Counter Narcan Could Save More Lives. But Price and Stigma Are Obstacles," *New York Times*, March 28, 2023.

19. C. Wesley Dunn, Federal Food, Drug, and Cosmetic Act, a Statement of its Legislative Record (New York: G. E. Stechert & Co., 1938), pp. 1083, 1195.

20. W. Steven Pray, *A History of Nonprescription Product Regulation* (Binghamton, NY: Pharmaceutical Products Press, 2003).

21. Singer and Cannon, "Drug Reformation," pp. 6–7.

22. Peter Barton Hutt, "A Legal Framework for Future Decisions on Transferring Drugs from Prescription to Nonprescription Status," *Food Drug Cosmetic Law Journal* 37 (1982): 428.

23. Sam Peltzman, "By Prescription Only ... or Occasionally?," *Regulation* 11, no. 3 (Fall/Winter 1987): 23–28.

24. Singer and Cannon, "Drug Reformation," pp. 6–7.

25. Singer and Cannon, "Drug Reformation," pp. 6–7.

26. Paul M. Wax, "Elixirs, Diluents, and the Passage of the 1938 Federal Food, Drug and Cosmetic Act," *Annals of Internal Medicine* 122, no. 6 (March 15, 1995): 456–61.

27. James Harvey Young, "Three Southern Food and Drug Cases," *Journal of Southern History* 49, no. 1 (February 1983): 3–36.

28. Jeffrey A. Singer, "End Government's Power to Require Prescriptions," *RealClearPolicy*, October 29, 2020.

29. Peter Temin, "The Origin of Compulsory Drug Prescriptions," *Journal of Law and Economics* 22, no. 1 (April 1979): 91–105.

30. Singer and Canon, "Drug Reformation," p. 8, quoting C. Wesley Dunn, *Federal Food, Drug, and Cosmetic Act, a Statement of its Legislative Record* (New York: G. E. Stechert & Co., 1938), p. 822.

31. Wax, "Passage of the 1938 Federal Food, Drug and Cosmetic Act."

32. Marra G. Katz et al., "Patient Literacy and Question-asking Behavior During the Medical Encounter: A Mixed-methods Analysis," *Journal of General Internal Medicine* 22, no. 6 (June 2007): 782–86.

33. Temin, "Origin of Compulsory Drug Prescriptions," p. 104.

34. Sam Peltzman, "The Health Effects of Mandatory Prescriptions," *Journal of Law and Economics* 30, no. 2 (October 1987): 207–38.

35. Solmaz Shotorbani et al., "Agreement between Women's and Providers' Assessment of Hormonal Contraceptive Risk Factors," *Contraception* 73, no. 5 (May 2006): 501–06.

36. Shotorbani et al., "Agreement," pp. 501–06; Jeffrey A. Singer, "End Government's Power to Require Prescriptions," *RealClearPolicy*, October 29, 2020; and Katie Thomas, "The Story of Thalidomide in the U.S., Told Through Documents," *New York Times*, March 23, 2020.

37. Harry M. Marks, "Revisiting 'The Origins of Compulsory Drug Prescriptions'," *American Journal of Public Health* 85, no. 1 (January 1995): 111.

38. Marks, "Revisiting 'The Origins of Compulsory Drug Prescriptions,'" p. 110.
39. Sam Peltzman, "The Health Effects of Mandatory Prescriptions," pp. 207–38.
40. Peltzman, "By Prescription Only . . . Or Occasionally?"
41. Jeffrey A. Singer and Michael F. Cannon, "Drug Reformation: End Government's Power to Require Prescriptions," Cato Institute White Paper, October 20, 2020, pp. 17–18.
42. "Motion Sickness," Aircraft Owners and Pilots Association.
43. Singer and Cannon, "Drug Reformation," pp. 25–31.
44. See Jonathan Anomaly, "How Should Antibiotics Be Regulated?," *Regulation* 42, no. 3 (Fall 2019): 18–21.
45. Singer and Cannon, "Drug Reformation," p. 36. For example, insulin and nitroglycerine are available over the counter in Canada; statin drugs, nitroglycerine, and sumatriptan are available over the counter in the United Kingdom; and asthma inhalers and nitroglycerine are available over the counter in Australia. Hormonal contraceptives are available over the counter in more than 100 countries. Tricia Tomiyoshi, "First Over-the-Counter Birth Control Pill Expected in Stores within Weeks: What Patients Need to Know," UC Davis Health News, March 6, 2024.
46. Sam Peltzman, "Prescription for Lower Drug Prices: More OTC Transitions," *Regulation* 41, no. 1 (Spring 2018): 2.
47. Singer and Cannon, "Drug Reformation," pp. 53–55.
48. Peltzman, "Prescription for Lower Drug Prices," p. 2.
49. Countries classifying certain drugs as behind-the-counter include the United Kingdom, Australia, the Netherlands, and Italy. "Nonprescrition Drugs: Considerations Regarding a Behind-the-Counter Drug Class," Government Accountability Office, GAO-09-245, February 2009.
50. Singer and Cannon, "Drug Reformation," p. 55.

Chapter 5

1. Jeffrey A. Singer and Michael F. Cannon, "Drug Reformation: End Government's Power to Require Prescriptions," Cato Institute White Paper, October 20, 2020, pp. 12–13.
2. Singer and Cannon, "Drug Reformation," pp. 12–13.
3. Suzanne White Junod, "FDA and Clinical Drug Trials: A Short History," US Food and Drug Administration, 2016, pp. 1–21.
4. Junod, "FDA and Clinical Drug Trials."
5. Hallie Levine, "How Seniors Can Save Money on Prescription Meds," *Consumer Reports*, December 5, 2022; and "Pharmacy Buying Guide," *Consumer Reports*, December 6, 2018.
6. J. Howard Beales III, "New Uses for Old Drugs," in *Competitive Strategies in the Pharmaceutical Industry*, ed. Robert B. Helms (Washington: American Enterprise Institute, 1996), pp. 281–305; and Singer and Cannon, "Drug Reformation," 49–50.
7. David C. Radley et al., "Off-Label Prescribing among Office-Based Physicians," *Archives of Internal Medicine* 166, no. 9 (May 8, 2006): 1021–26.

8. Harry M. Marks, *The Progress of Experiment: Science and Therapeutic Reform in the United States, 1900–1990* (Cambridge, MA: Cambridge University Press, 2000) p. 82, citing Henry O. Calvery and Theodore G. Klumpp, "The Toxicity for Human Beings of Diethylene Glycol with Sulfanilamide," *Southern Medical Journal* 32 (1939): 1106–07.

9. Public Health and Welfare, 42 U.S.C. § 1395x(t)(2)(B)(ii)(I).

10. The secretary has designated the following additional compendia and journals as authoritative sources of efficacy certification of anticancer drugs: Micromedex DrugDex (successor to the USP-DI); the Clinical Pharmacology compendium; the Wolters Kluwer Lexi-Drugs compendium; and the National Comprehensive Cancer Network Drugs and Biologics Compendium; *American Journal of Medicine; Annals of Internal Medicine; Annals of Oncology; Annals of Surgical Oncology; Biology of Blood and Marrow Transplantation; Blood; Bone Marrow Transplantation; British Journal of Cancer; British Journal of Haematology; British Medical Journal; Cancer; Clinical Cancer Research; Clinical Cancer Drugs; European Journal of Cancer; Gynecologic Oncology; International Journal of Radiation Oncology, Biology, Physics; Journal of the American Medical Association; Journal of Clinical Oncology; Journal of the National Cancer Institute; Journal of the National Comprehensive Cancer Network; Journal of Urology; Lancet; Lancet Oncology; Leukemia; New England Journal of Medicine;* and *Radiation Oncology.* Public Health and Welfare, 42 U.S.C. § 1395x(t)(2)(B)(ii)(I); "Recent Developments in Medicare Coverage of Off-Label Cancer Therapies," *Journal of Oncology Practice* 5, no. 1 (January 2009): 18–20; and "Wolters Kluwer Clinical Drug Information Lexi-Drugs Compendium Revision Request—CAG-00443O," Centers for Medicare and Medicaid Services, April 21, 2015.

11. Federal law requires state Medicaid programs to cover off-label uses of drugs that are found in the "American Hospital Formulary Service Drug Information; United States Pharmacopeia-Drug Information (or its successor publications); [the] DRUGDEX Information System; and the peer-reviewed medical literature." Public Health and Welfare, 42 U.S.C. §§ 1396r–8(d)(1) (B)(i), (g)(1)(B)(i), and (k)(6).

12. Singer and Cannon, "Drug Reformation," 49–50.

13. Sam Kazman, "Drug Approvals and Deadly Delays," *Journal of American Physicians and Surgeons* 15 no. 4 (Winter 2010): 101–03. For example, the FDA delayed approving beta-blockers, which are crucial to treating high blood pressure and reducing heart attack risk and had been approved in Europe, and interleukin-2, which is used to treat kidney cancer and had been approved in nine European countries.

14. Singer and Cannon, "Drug Reformation," 13–14.

15. Right to Try; and Rachel Roubein, "House Approves 'Right to Try,' Sends Bill to Trump's Desk," *The Hill*, May 22, 2018.

16. "Patient Stories," Right to Try.

17. Joanne Kenen, "How Testing Failures Allowed Coronavirus to Sweep the U.S.," *Politico*, March 6, 2020; Carolyn Y. Johnson and Laurie McGinley, "What Went Wrong with the Coronavirus Tests in the U.S.," *Washington Post*, March 7, 2020; and Jeffrey A. Singer, "Coronavirus Testing Delays Caused by Red Tape, Bureaucracy and Scorn for Private Companies," *NBC News*, March 18, 2020.

18. Stephen Engelberg, Lisa Song, and Lydia DePillis, "How South Korea Scaled Coronavirus Testing While the U.S. Fell Dangerously Behind," *ProPublica*, March 15, 2020; Jon Cohen, "The United States Badly Bungled Coronavirus Testing—But Things May Soon Improve," *Science*, February 28, 2020; and Stefan Nicola, "A Berlin Biotech Company Got a Head Start on Coronavirus Tests," Bloomberg, March 12, 2020.

19. Laurie McGinley, Carolyn Y. Johnson, and William Wan, "New FDA Policy Will Expand Coronavirus Testing," *Washington Post*, February 29, 2020; "Policy for Diagnostics Testing in Laboratories Certified to Perform High Complexity Testing under CLIA Prior to Emergency Use Authorization for Coronavirus Disease-2019 during the Public Health Emergency Immediately in Effect Guidance for Clinical Laboratories and Food and Drug Administration Staff," US Food and Drug Administration, Regulations.gov; and Steven H. Woolf et al., "Excess Deaths From COVID-19 and Other Causes, March-April 2020," *JAMA*, July 1, 2020.

20. "Coronavirus (COVID-19) Update: FDA Authorizes First COVID-19 Test for Self-Testing at Home," US Food and Drug Administration, press release, November 17, 2020; "FDA Authorizes the First Prescription At-Home COVID-19 Test Kit," Optum, November 24, 2020; Jeffrey A. Singer, "A Prescription Is Not Required for an At-Home Pregnancy Test or an At-Home HIV Test—Why Require One for an At-Home COVID Test?," *Cato at Liberty* (blog), Cato Institute, November 18, 2020; "Coronavirus (COVID-19) Update: FDA Issues New Authorization for the BinaxNOW COVID-19 Ag Card Home Test," US Food and Drug Administration, December 16, 2020; and "Coronavirus (COVID-19) Update: FDA Authorizes Antigen Test as First Over-the-Counter Fully At-Home Diagnostic Test for COVID-19," US Food and Drug Administration, December 15, 2020.

21. Karla Adam and Niha Masih, "Free Rapid Tests Are About to Roll out in the U.S. In other Countries, They're Already Part of Daily Life," *Washington Post*, January 20, 2022.

22. Shelby Baird, "Don't Try This at Home: The FDA's Restrictive Regulations of Home-Testing Devices," *Duke Law Journal* 67 (2017): 383–426.

23. Baird, "Don't Try This at Home," p. 392n46.

24. Baird, "Don't Try This at Home," pp. 398–404.

25. Baird, "Don't Try This at Home," pp. 404–10.

26. "Survey of Direct-to-Consumer Testing Statutes and Regulations," Genetics and Public Policy Center, Berman Institute of Bioethics, Johns Hopkins University, June 2007.

27. For a discussion of the FDA's incentives to favor delay over access to drugs, see Michael F. Cannon, "Health Care Regulation," in *Cato Handbook for Policymakers*, 9th ed. (Washington: Cato Institute, 2022).

28. Nicole C. Perez, "International Reciprocity: If a Drug Is Good Enough for Great Britain, It Should Be Good Enough for the United States," *University of Miami Business Law Review* 25, no. 1 (2016): 169–93; and Jeffrey A. Singer, "The Economic Impact of America's Failure to Contain the Coronavirus," Cato Institute, September 22, 2020.

29. Christian Johner "CE Marking for Medical Devices: Is there a CE Certification?," Johner Institute, December 9, 2015; and "The European Regulatory System for Medicines," European Medicines Agency, 2023.

30. "Regulation," Pharma Israel.

31. Anita Holler, "Politicians Decide in Favour of Patient Care," Swiss Medtech, November 28, 2022.

32. Nick Paul Taylor, "Australia Starts Accepting FDA Reports in Device Filings," *MedTech Dive*, August 22, 2018.

33. The FDA did not approve some drugs because the manufacturers never submitted or withdrew them. Some drugs posed such significant risks that regulators withdrew approval. Only 4 out of 10 novel drugs without therapeutic alternatives had their initial applications rejected by the FDA. The remaining 6 were either approved on the first submission (3), withdrawn by the sponsor before evaluation (2), or never submitted (1). Of 37 novel drugs approved outside the United States, the FDA rejected 19 on their first submission, of which 12 were rejected for safety reasons. Only 4 of these rejected drugs were for indications without approved therapies in the United States, with 3 for orphan diseases. Of the 12 drugs initially rejected for safety reasons, the FDA eventually approved 9, while 2—laropiprant/nicotinic acid (Pelzont) and rimonabant (Acomplia)—were withdrawn from the European market due to safety concerns. Matthieu Larochelle et al., "Assessing the Potential Clinical Impact of Reciprocal Drug Approval Legislation on Access to Novel Therapeutics in the USA: a Cohort Study," *British Medical Journal Open* 7, no. e014582 (2017): 2–3. Even so, if a drug is available in another developed country, the FDA's premarket approval requirement denies consumers, many of whom will have a greater tolerance for risk than the FDA, the freedom to make their own medical decisions.

34. See, for example: "Misplaced Trust: Why FDA Approval Does Not Guarantee Drug Safety," Drugwatch.

Chapter 6

1. Lily Rothman, "The History of Poisoned Alcohol in America Includes an Unlikely Culprit: The U.S. Government," *Time*, January 14, 2015.

2. "21st Amendment Is Ratified; Prohibition Ends," This Day in History, History. com, last updated December 4, 2023; and Stephen Lusk, "Alcohol Prohibition Isn't Dead in Mississippi," Foundation for Economic Education March 17, 2018.

3. E. M. Brecher, "Drug Laws and Drug Law Enforcement: A Review and Evaluation Based on 111 Years of Experience," *Drugs and Society* 1, no. 1 (Fall 1986): 1–27.

4. Kat Eschner, "Why the Ku Klux Klan Flourished Under Prohibition," *Smithsonian*, December 5, 2017.

5. Jacob Sullum, "Anti-Chinese Xenophobia Fueled America's First Drug War," *Reason*, May 2024.

6. Edward Huntington Williams, "Negro Cocaine 'Fiends' Are a New Southern Menace," *New York Times*, February 8, 1914; and Carl L. Hart, "How the Myth

of the 'Negro Cocaine Fiend' Helped Shape American Drug Policy," *The Nation*, January 29, 2014.

7. Eric Schlosser, "Reefer Madness," *The Atlantic*, August 1994.

8. Dan Baum, "Legalize It All: How to Win the War on Drugs," *Harper's Magazine*, April 2016.

9. Benjamin T. Smith, "New Documents Reveal the Bloody Origins of America's Long War on Drugs," *Time*, August 24, 2021.

10. Jeffrey A. Singer, and Trevor Burrus, "Cops Practicing Medicine: The Parallel Histories of Drug War I and Drug War II," Cato Institute White Paper, November 29, 2022.

11. "Provisional Drug Overdose Data," National Center for Health Statistics, Centers for Disease Control and Prevention.

12. Hawre Jalal et al., "Changing Dynamics of the Drug Overdose Epidemic in the United States from 1979 through 2016," *Science* 361, no. 6408, (September 21, 2018): aau1184.

13. "Long-Term Trends in Deaths of Despair," United States Congress Joint Economic Committee, September 5, 2019.

14. Lori Ann Post et al., "Geographic Trends in Opioid Overdoses in the US from 1999 to 2020," *JAMA Network Open* 5, no. 7 (July 28, 2022): e2223631.

15. Jeffrey A. Singer, "An Encouraging Report on Overdose Deaths," *Cato at Liberty* (blog), Cato Institute, September 18, 2024; "Provisional Drug Overdose Death Counts," Centers for Disease control and Prevention, National Center for Health Statistics, updated August 18, 2024; and Brian Mann, "NPR Exclusive: U.S. Overdose Deaths Plummet, Saving Thousands of Lives," NPR, September 18, 2024.

16. "Prescription Opioid Trends in the United States," IQVIA Institute for Human Data Science, December 16, 2020; Jeffrey A. Singer, "An Encouraging Report on Overdose Deaths," *Cato at Liberty* (blog), Cato Institute, September 18, 2024; "Provisional Drug Overdose Death Counts," US Centers for Disease Control and Prevention, National Center for Health Statistics, updated August 18, 2024; and Brian Mann, "NPR Exclusive: U.S. Overdose Deaths Plummet, Saving Thousands of Lives," NPR, September 18, 2024.

17. "DEA Proposes to Reduce the Amount of Five Opioids Manufactured in 2020, Marijuana Quota for Research Increases by almost a Third," Drug Enforcement Administration, news release, September 11, 2019; and Jeffrey A. Singer, "Is the DEA Branching Out into Regulating Medicine?," *Cato At Liberty* (blog), Cato Institute, September 23, 2019.

18. Jeffrey A. Singer, Jacob Z. Sullum, and Michael E. Schatman, "Today's Nonmedical Opioid Users Are Not Yesterday's Patients; Implications of Data Indicating Stable Rates of Nonmedical Use and Pain Reliever Use Disorder," *Journal of Pain Research* 12 (February 2019): 617–20; "Results from the 2014 National Survey on Drug Use and Health: Detailed Tables," Substance Abuse and Mental Health Services Administration, 2015, Table 6.47.

19. Robert Capodilupo and Jacob James Rich, "The Misinformed and Misguided Prescription Abuse Prevention Act: A Response to Delfino," *Yale Law and Policy Review* (Spring 2023): 5.

20. "Are Fentanyl Overdose Deaths Rising in the US?," USA Facts, updated September 27, 2023.

21. "Unintentional Drug Poisoning (Overdose) Deaths in New York City, 2000 to 2017," *NYC Health, Epi Data Brief*, no. 104, September 2018.

22. "Unintentional Drug Poisoning," NYC Health.

23. Singer et al., "Today's Nonmedical Opioid Users Are not Yesterday's Patients," pp. 617–20.

24. "Desoxyn—Uses, Side Effects, and More," WebMD.

25. "Meth Epidemic," Department of Justice, Office of Justice Programs, 2006.

26. "Combat Methamphetamine Epidemic Act of 2005 (CMEA): Preventing the Retail Diversion of Pseudoephedrine," Department of Justice, Drug Enforcement Administration, Office of Diversion Control, 2008.

27. Conor Radnovich, "Pseudoephedrine Products Now Available in Oregon without Prescription," *Statesman Journal*, January 1, 2022; "Mississippi Law Erases Prescription for Some Decongestants," AP News, December 31, 2021.

28. "Combat Methamphetamine Epidemic Act of 2005," Department of Justice.

29. Ronald Eccles, "Substitution of Phenylephrine for Pseudoephedrine as a Nasal Decongeststant. An Illogical Way to Control Methamphetamine Abuse," *British Journal of Clinical Pharmacology* 63, no. 1 (2006): 10–14; and Isabella Backman, "Phenylephrine, a Common Decongestant, Is Ineffective, Say FDA Advisors. It's Not Alone," Yale School of Medicine, October 5, 2023.

30. Berkeley Lovelace Jr., "FDA Panel Says Common Over-the-Counter Decongestant Doesn't Work," *NBC News*, September 12, 2023.

31. "The Rise of Super Meth: The Destructive Effects of P2P Methamphetamine," PharmChek, February 14, 2023.

32. "Data Brief 428. Drug Overdose Deaths in the United States, 1999–2020," Centers for Disease Control and Prevention, National Center for Health Statistics; and Jeffrey A. Singer, "FDA Says the Decongestant in Your Medicine Cabinet Probably Doesn't Work. Now What?," *USA Today*, October 25, 2023.

33. Michael Shifter, "Plan Colombia: A Retrospective," *Americas Quarterly*, July 18, 2012.

34. Ted Galen Carpenter and Jeffrey Singer, "We Shouldn't Use the Military to Fight Mexico's Drug Cartels," *Daily Beast*, April 3, 2023; and Mark Gollom, "Why the Arrest of El Chapo's Son Caused a Rampage of Violence in a Mexican City," CBC News, January 6, 2023.

35. Mike Riggs, "Illegal Drugs Are Cheaper and More Pure than Ever," Bloomberg, October 1, 2013.

36. "Drug Overdose Deaths," Centers for Disease Control and Prevention, last reviewed August 22, 2023.

37. "History of Cannabis," Lambert Initiative for Cannabinoid Therapeutics, University of Sydney.

38. Christopher J. Boes, "Osler on Migraine," *Canadian Journal of Neurological Sciences* 42, no. 2 (2015): 144–47; Michelle Sexton and Nathaniel M. Schuster, "Medical Cannabis for Migraine and Pain," *Practical Neurology*, May 2021.

39. "Drug Scheduling," Drug Enforcement Administration.

40. Nick Wing, "Marijuana Prohibition Was Racist from the Start. Not Much Has Changed.," *Huffington Post*, January 14, 2014.

41. "Did You Know . . . Marijuana Was Once a Legal Cross-Border Import?," US Customs and Border Protection; and David F. Musto, "The Marihuana Tax Act of 1937," *Archives of General Psychiatry* 26, no. 2 (1972): 101–08.

42. David Downs, "The Science behind the DEA's Long War on Marijuana," *Scientific American*, April 19, 2016.

43. "A Tale of Two Countries: Racially Targeted Arrests in the Era of Marijuana Reform," American Civil Liberties Union, April 16, 2020.

44. Tara García Mathewson, "Licensing Barriers Keep People with Criminal Records from Education and Training," *Washington Post*, August 6, 2023. Several state medical licensing boards will revoke the licenses of physicians convicted of felonies. "Limits on Use of Criminal Record in Licensing, State-by-State Overview," Federation of State Medical Boards.

45. Petter Grahl Johnstad, "Comparative Harms Assessments for Cannabis, Alcohol, and Tobacco: Risk for Psychosis, Cognitive Impairment, and Traffic Accident," *Drug Science, Policy and Law* 8 (2022).

46. Dave Dormer, "Why Overdose May Be the Wrong Word When It Comes to Cannabis," *CBC News*, September 10, 2018.

47. E. B. De Sousa et al., "Subjective Aggression during Alcohol and Cannabis Intoxication before and after Aggression Exposure," *Psychopharmacology* 233 (2016): 3331–40.

48. Cornelis Jan van Dam et al., "Inhaled Δ^9-tetrahydrocannabinol Does Not Enhance Oxycodone-Induced Respiratory Depression: Randomised Controlled Trial in Healthy Volunteers," *British Journal of Anaesthesia* 130, no. 4 (2023): 485–93.

49. Preeti Vankar, "Marijuana Use among U.S. Adults within the past Year 2022 by State," Statista, March 8, 2024.

50. Lydia Saad, "Grassroots Support for Legalizing Marijuana Hits Record 70%," Gallup, November 8, 2023.

51. "State Medical Cannabis Laws," National Conference of State Legislatures, updated June 4, 2024.

52. "State Medical Cannabis Laws." Although District of Columbia voters legalized recreational marijuana in 2014, Congress banned marijuana sales in the District. To get around this obstruction, marijuana dealers have devised a mechanism whereby they sell an unrelated item to a customer and give them marijuana as a gift with the purchase. Katie Sheppard, "The Difference between Buying Weed in D.C., Maryland and Virginia," *Washington Post*, May 3, 2023.

53. "Presidential Proclamation on Marijuana Possession, Attempted Possession, and Use," Office of the Pardon Attorney, US Department of Justice; and Jeffrey A. Singer, "Marijuana Should Be De-Scheduled, Not Re-Scheduled," *Cato at Liberty* (blog), Cato Institute, August 30, 2023.

54. Christina Jewett and Noah Weiland, "Federal Scientists Recommend Easing Restrictions on Marijuana," *New York Times*, January 12, 2024.

55. "DEA Drug Scheduling," Drug Enforcement Administration.

56. Jewett and Weiland, "Federal Scientists Recommend Easing Restrictions."

57. Zeke Miller et al., "US Poised to Ease Restrictions on Marijuana in Historic Shift, But It'll Remain Controlled Substance," Associated Press, April 30, 2024.

58. Jeffrey A. Singer, "Beer, Wine, Whiskey, Cigars, and Cigarettes Are Not on the DEA's List of Controlled Substances. Neither Should Cannabis Be," *Cato at Liberty* (blog), Cato Institute, April 30, 2024; and Jacob Sullum, "Rescheduling Marijuana Does Not Address Today's Central Cannabis Issue," *Reason*, May 1, 2024.

59. David E. Nichols, "Psychedelics," *Pharmacological Reviews* 68, no. 2 (2016): 264–355.

60. "FDA Warns Patients and Health Care Providers about Potential Risks Associated with Compounded Ketamine Products," US Food and Drug Administration, last modified October 10, 2023.

61. "FDA Approves New Nasal Spray Medication for Treatment-Resistant Depression; Available Only at a Certified Doctor's Office or Clinic," US Food and Drug Administration, March 5, 2019.

62. Joseph J. Palamar, Caroline Rutherford, and Katherine M. Keyes, "Trends in Ketamine Use, Exposures, and Seizures in the United States up to 2019," *American Journal of Public Health* 111, no. 11 (November 1, 2021): 2046–49.

63. Brian Pilecki et al., "Ethical and Legal Issues in Psychedelic Harm Reduction and Integration Therapy," *Harm Reduction Journal* 18, no. 40 (2021).

64. "U.S. Will Ban Ecstasy, a Hallucinogenic Drug," *New York Times*, June 1, 1985.

65. Jamie Ducharme, "Psychedelics May Be Part of U.S. Medicine Sooner Than You Think," *Time*, February 8, 2023; Rachel Nuwer, "MDMA Therapy Inches Closer to Approval," *New York Times*, September 14, 2023; "FDA Issues First Draft Guidance on Clinical Trials with Psychedelic Drugs," US Food and Drug Administration, FDA news release, June 23, 2023; and Berkeley Lovelace Jr., "FDA Panel Rejects First MDMA Treatment Amid Deep Concerns About Flawed Trials," NBC News, June 4, 2024.

66. Madison Carlino, "The Latest on Proposed Psychedelics Legalization in States," Reason Foundation, April 13, 2023; Jeffrey A. Singer, "Governor Newsom Bars Californians from Self-Medicating with Psychedelics," *Cato at Liberty* (blog), Cato Institute, October 9, 2023.

67. See for example Jessica J. Fulton et al., "The Prevalence of Posttraumatic Stress Disorder in Operation Enduring Freedom/Operation Iraqi Freedom (OEF/OIF) Veterans: a Meta-Analysis," *Journal of Anxiety Disorders* (April 2015): 98–107; and Erik Eng Berge, Roger Hagen, and Joar Øveraas Halvorsen, "PTSD Relapse in Veterans of Iraq and Afghanistan: A Systematic Review," *Military Psychology* 32 no. 4 (2020): 300–12.

68. Richard Cowan, "How the Narcs Created Crack," *National Review* 38 no. 23 (December 5, 1986): 26–34; Junichi Minagawa and Thorsten Upmann, "The Generalized Alchian–Allen Theorem: A Slutsky Equation for Relative Demand," *Economic Inquiry* 53, no. 4 (October 2015): 1893–1907. Armen A. Alchian and William R. Allen were prominent academic economists who coauthored several works, including *University Economics*, an influential textbook in 1964. See also Sarah Beller, "Infographic: The Iron Law of Prohibition," *Filter*, October 3, 2018.

69. Kavita Babu, "What is Xylazine? A Medical Toxicologist Explains," UMass Chan Medical School, March 31, 2023.

70. Babu, "What is Xylazine?"

71. J. C. Reyes et al., "The Emerging of Xylazine as a New Drug of Abuse and Its Health Consequences among Drug Users in Puerto Rico," *Journal of Urban Health* 89, no. 3 (June 1, 2012): 519–26.

72. J. M. Bowles et al., "Xylazine Detected in Unregulated Opioids and Drug Administration Equipment in Toronto, Canada: Clinical and Social Implications," *Harm Reduction Journal* 18, no. 104 (2021); and "Xylazine Circulating in Toronto's Unregulated Drug Supply," Drug Checking Community.

73. "DEA Reports Widespread Threat of Fentanyl Mixed with Xylazine," Drug Enforcement Administration.

74. Allison Roberts, Jessica Korona-Bailey, and Sutapa Mukhopadhyay, "*Notes from the Field*: Nitazene-Related Deaths—Tennessee, 2019–2021," Centers for Disease Control and Prevention, Morbidity and Mortality Weekly Report, September 16, 2022.

75. "Synthetic Opioids: Largest Ever UK Seizure Made by Police," BBC News, November 23, 2023; Amy-Clare Martin, Tara Cobham, and Rebecca Thomas, "Is the UK Sleepwalking into a Lethal US-style Opioid Drugs Crisis?," *The Independent*, December 26, 2023; and Jeffrey A. Singer, "Unfortunately, as I Warned Lawmakers in March, We May Soon Be Talking about the Nitazene Crisis," *Cato at Liberty* (blog), Cato Institute, December 28, 2023.

76. Nora D. Volkow and A. Thomas McLellan, "Opioid Abuse in Chronic Pain—Misconceptions and Mitigation Strategies," *New England Journal of Medicine* 374, no 13. (March 31, 2016): 1253–63; Gavan P. McNally et al., "Pathways to the Persistence of Drug Use Despite Its Adverse Consequences," *Molecular Psychiatry* 28 (2023): 2228–37; and Jeffrey A. Singer, "The March toward a Pre-Modern Approach to the Treatment of Pain Continues, Undeterred by Science," *Cato at Liberty* (blog), Cato Institute, August 12, 2019.

77. "What Is Gambling Disorder?," American Psychiatric Association, last reviewed August 2021.

78. Gina B. Polychronopoulos et al., "The Emergence of Behavioral Addiction in DSM-5," *Journal of Human Services* 34, no. 1 (2014): 20; and M. Piquet-Pessôa, G. M. Ferreira, I. A. Melca, et al., "DSM-5 and the Decision Not to Include Sex, Shopping or Stealing as Addictions," *Current Addict Reports* 1 (2014): 172–76.

79. Shane Darke, Sarah Larney, and Michael Farrell, "Yes, People Can Die from Opiate Withdrawal," National Drug and Alcohol Research Center, University of New South Wales.

80. Kurt W. Prins et al., "Effects of Beta-Blocker Withdrawal in Acute Decompensated Heart Failure: A Systematic Review and Meta-Analysis," *JACC: Heart Failure* 3, no. 8 (2015): 647–53.

81. "Cocaine Withdrawal," MedlinePlus, US National Library of Medicine, updated January 2, 2023; and Todd Zorick et al., "Withdrawal Symptoms in Abstinent Methamphetamine-Dependent Subjects," *Addiction* 105, no. 10 (2010): 1809–18.

82. Lamya Khoury et al., "Substance Use, Childhood Traumatic Experience, and Posttraumatic Stress Disorder in an Urban Civilian Population," *Depression*

and Anxiety 27, no. 12 (December 2010): 1077–86; "Making the Connection: Trauma and Substance Abuse," National Child Traumatic Stress Network, June 2008; and Amanda L. Giordano, "Why Trauma Can Lead to Addiction," *Psychology Today*, September 25, 2021.

83. "Common Comorbidities with Substance Use Disorders Research Report," National Institute on Drug Abuse, April 2020; and Substance Abuse and Mental Health Services Administration, "Obsessive-Compulsive Disorder and Substance Use Disorders," *Advisory* 15, no. 3 (Fall 2016).

84. Maia Szalavitz, "Genetics: No More Addictive Personality," *Nature* 522 (2015): S48–S49.

85. D. A. Nielsen et al., "Epigenetics of Drug Abuse: Predisposition or Response," *Pharmacogenomics* 13, no. 10 (July 2012): 1149–60.

86. Nora D. Volkow and A. Thomas McLellan, "Opioid Abuse in Chronic Pain—Misconceptions and Mitigation Strategies," *New England Journal of Medicine* 374, no. 13 (March 31, 2016): 1253–63.

87. Katherine Schaeffer, "9 Facts about Americans and Marijuana," Pew Research Center, April 10, 2024.

Chapter 7

1. Luca Paoletti et al., "Current Status of Tobacco Policy and Control," *Journal of Thoracic Imaging* 27, no. 4 (July 2012): 213–19.

2. Cassandra Tate, *Cigarette Wars: The Triumph of "The Little White Slaver"* (New York: Oxford University Press, 2000), p. 5. The judge sentenced smoker Jenny Lasher for endangering the lives of her children by smoking in their presence after her husband brought the complaint. A contemporary newspaper account noted that "the conviction is the first of its kind under the New York State law." "Jail for Smoking Mother," *Rock Island Argus*, November 5, 1904.

3. Erin Blakemore, "When New York Banned Smoking to Save Women's Souls," History.com, updated May 23, 2023.

4. Jeremy Richards, "History Shows Smoking Bans Likely to Be Repealed," Heartland Institute, July 1, 2008.

5. Dan Glaister, "'My Voice Is Clear as a Bell in Every Scene!' How Big Tobacco Bought the Big Screen," *The Guardian*, September 25, 2008.

6. Becky Little, "When Cigarette Companies Used Doctors to Push Smoking," History.com, updated March 28, 2023.

7. "The 1964 Report on Smoking and Health," Reports of the Surgeon General, National Library of Medicine.

8. Jeffrey M. Jones, "U.S. Cigarette Smoking Rate Steady Near Historical Low," Gallup, August 18, 2023.

9. "Youth Data," Smoking and Tobacco Use, US Centers for Disease Control and Prevention, last reviewed November 2, 2023.

10. This oft-quoted saying is of uncertain provenance, though it has been attributed to various individuals, from Justice Oliver Wendell Holmes to Abraham Lincoln. "Your Liberty to Swing Your Fist Ends Just where My Nose Begins," Quote Investigator, October 15, 2011.

11. Ronald Bayer, "Tobacco, Commercial Speech, and Libertarian Values: the End of the Line for Restrictions on Advertising?" *American Journal of Public Health* 92, no. 3 (March 1, 2002): 356–59; and Garrett Epps, "Does Cigarette Marketing Count as Free Speech?," *The Atlantic*, August 29, 2012.

12. "The Master Settlement Agreement," National Association of Attorneys General. Terms of the settlement agreement included a ban on advertising targeting youth and on advertising and labeling that uses cartoons, imposing payment obligations on tobacco companies that would raise the price of their products, and establishing and funding the "Truth Initiative," a project seeking to change culture to make tobacco unattractive to youth.

13. Kashish Aneja and Sanjana Gopal, "Bhutan Reverses Sales Ban on Tobacco," *Tobacco Control* (blog), British Medical Journal, February 1, 2023.

14. "Bhutan Tops Tobacco and Marijuana Users in South East Asia," Kuensel, July 4, 2017.

15. Karen Evans-Reeves, "Bhutan Reverses Sales Ban on Tobacco," *BMJ Tobacco Control Blog*, February 1, 2023.

16. "Health Experts Decry New Zealand's Scrapping of World-First Tobacco Ban," Reuters, November 28, 2023; and "New Zealand Smoking Rate 1960–2024," Macrotrends.

17. "Britain Proposes Ban on Cigarettes for Younger Generations," Reuters, October 4, 2023.

18. Duarte Dias, "U.K. Lawmakers Back Anti-smoking Bill, Moving Step Closer to a Future Ban on All Tobacco Sales," CBS News, April 17, 2024.

19. Patrick Lagreid, "Brookline, Mass.'s Tobacco Sales Ban Survives Court Challenge," Halfwheel, November 2, 2022.

20. Daniela Pardo and Jackson Ellison, "California Bill Would Phase Out Tobacco Sales for Future Generations," *Spectrum News 1*, March 2, 2023.

21. Alexei Koseff, " Tobacco Sales Phaseout Withers in California without Support from Tobacco Advocates," *CalMatters*, April 13, 2023.

22. Jacob James Rich and Jordan Campbell, "The Effect of Menthol Bans on Cigarette Sales: Evidence from Massachusetts," Reason Foundation, February 15, 2023.

23. Adam Hoffer, "Californians Still Smoking Menthol after Ban: Evidence from a Discarded Pack Audit," Tax Foundation, October 26, 2023.

24. Klaus von Lampe, Marin Kurti, and Jacqueline Johnson, " 'I'm Gonna Get Me a Loosie' Understanding Single Cigarette Purchases by Adult Smokers in a Disadvantaged Section of New York City," *Preventive Medicine Reports* 12 (December 2018): 182–85.

25. Jacob Sullum, "It Wasn't Just a Chokehold That Killed Eric Garner," *Reason*, August 21, 2019.

26. Sullum, "It Wasn't Just a Chokehold That Killed Eric Garner."

27. Adam Hoffer, "State Cigarette Taxes and Cigarette Smuggling by State, 2020," Tax Foundation, December 6, 2022.

28. "Youth Data," Centers for Disease Control and Prevention, November 2, 2023.

29. Andrea S. Gentzke et al., "Tobacco Product Use and Associated Factors among Middle and High School Students—National Youth Tobacco Survey, United States, 2021," *MMWR Surveillance Summaries* 71, no. 5 (2022): 1–29.

30. Guy Bentley and Jacob James Rich, "Does Menthol Cigarette Distribution Affect Child or Adult Cigarette Use?," Reason Foundation, January 30, 2020.

31. David Janazzo, "EU Menthol Cigarette Ban Survey," Global Action to End Smoking, January 28, 2021; and Anne-Line Brink, Andrea Stadil Glahn, and Niels Them Kjaer, "Tobacco Companies' Exploitation of Loopholes in the EU Ban on Menthol Cigarettes: A Case Study from Denmark," *Tobacco Control* 32, no. 6 (2023): 809.

32. Alan Selby, "Gangs Are Making Millions Smuggling Menthol Cigarettes to Beat an EU Ban," *Mirror*, July 28, 2020.

33. Jeffrey A. Singer, "Expect Ban on Menthol Cigarettes to Worsen Inequities in Criminal Justice," *Orange County Register*, May 6, 2021.

34. Jeffrey A. Singer, "Public Comments on FDA's Proposed Tobacco Product Standard That Would Prohibit Menthol as a Characterizing Flavor in Cigarettes," Cato Institute, May 4, 2022.

35. Dan Diamond and David Ovalle, "Biden Ban on Menthol Cigarettes to be Delayed Amid Political Concerns, Officials Say," *Washington Post*, December 6, 2023.

36. "Secretary Becerra Statement on the Proposed Menthol Cigarette Rule," Department of Health and Human Services, press release, April 26, 2024; and Jeffrey A. Singer, "Biden Administration Again Delays Decision on Banning Menthol Tobacco," *Cato at Liberty* (blog), Cato Institute, April 29, 2024.

37. William J. Blot et al., "Lung Cancer Risk among Smokers of Menthol Cigarettes," *Journal of the National Cancer Institute* 103, no. 10 (March 23, 2011): 810–16.

38. Brian Rostron, "Lung Cancer Mortality Risk for U.S. Menthol Cigarette Smokers," *Nicotine & Tobacco Research* 14, no. 10 (October 2012): 1140–44.

39. Heather M Munro et al., "Smoking Quit Rates among Menthol vs Nonmenthol Smokers: Implications Regarding a US Ban on the Sale of Menthol Cigarettes," *Journal of the National Cancer Institute* 114, no. 7 (April 2022): 953.

40. Parker Beene, "Recent Federal and State Actions to Limit Flavored Tobacco Products," Association of State and Territorial Health Officials, March 2, 2023; and Nada Hassanein, "States Consider Menthol Cigarette Bans as Feds Delay Action," Stateline, February 29, 2024.

Chapter 8

1. Mike Moen, "Adolescents' Tech Addiction Is a Growing Problem, Therapists Say," *NPR*, June 17, 2019; Sam Kerrigan, "Experts Warn Social Media May Be Highly Addictive to Young Minds," *CBS12 News*, February 10, 2023; and Luis Velarde, "How Addictive, Endless Scrolling is Bad for Your Mental Health," *Washington Post*, July 14, 2023.

2. *Open Hearing on Foreign Influence Operations' Use of Social Media Platforms (Company Witnesses), Hearing Before the Select Committee on Intelligence,* 115th Cong. 2nd Sess. (September 5, 2018); and "Lawmakers Examine Addictive Powers of Social Media," *Fox News,* September 6, 2018.

3. Charles Hymas, "Facebook 'Founder' Claims Social Media Site Has 'Caused Countless Deaths by Failing to Protect Users,'" *The Telegraph* (London), August 28, 2018.

4. Jeffrey A. Singer, "The Panic over 'Social Media Addiction' Threatens Free Speech," *Reason,* April 23, 2019; and Jeffrey A. Singer, "Stop Saying Social Media 'Addiction,'" *MedPage Today,* September 20, 2018.

5. Laura J. Felt and Michael B. Robb, "Technology Addiction: Concern, Controversy, and Finding Balance," *Common Sense Media,* May 2016.

6. "Conditions for Further Study," in *Diagnostic and Statistical Manual of Mental Disorders,* 5th ed. (Washington: American Psychiatric Association, 2013; and Ronald Pies, "Should DSM-V Designate 'Internet Addiction' a Mental Disorder?" *Psychiatry (Edgmont)* 6, no. 2 (February 2009): 31–37.

7. Daria J. Kuss and Mark D. Griffiths, "Online Social Networking and Addiction—A Review of the Psychological Literature," *International Journal of Environmental Research and Public Health* 8, no. 9 (August 2011): 3528–52.

8. Daria J. Kuss and Mark D. Griffiths, "Social Networking Sites and Addiction: Ten Lessons Learned," *International Journal of Environmental Research and Public Health* 14, no. 3 (March 2017): 311.

9. Madelyn Brown, "Does Social Media Cause Depression?," *Psych Central,* March 7, 2022; and Amy Orben, "Social Media and Suicide: A Critical Appraisal," *Medium,* November 14, 2017.

10. Clare Foran, "The Rise of the Internet-Addiction Industry," *The Atlantic,* November 5, 2015.

11. Barbara Booth, "Internet Addiction Is Sweeping America, Affecting Millions," CNBC, August 29, 2017.

12. "Addictive Behaviours: Gaming Disorder," World Health Organization, October 22, 2020. Contrary to the World Health Organization, the American Psychiatric Association classifies "internet gaming disorder" as a condition "warranting more clinical research and experience" before including it in the *Diagnostic and Statistical Manual of Mental Disorders* as a formal disorder. "Internet Gaming Disorder," American Psychiatric Association.

13. Rachel Williams, "China Recognizes Internet Addiction as a New Disease," *The Guardian* (London), November 11, 2008.

14. Wu Peiyue, "Inside China's Brutal Internet Addiction Clinics," *Sixth Tone,* October 21, 2022.

15. Robert van Voren, "Political Abuse of Psychiatry—An Historical Overview," *Schizophrenia Bulletin* 36 no. 1 (2010): 33–35.

16. "Japan to Start Internet Fasting Camps for Web Addicted Kids," *Hindustan Times,* August 28, 2013; and Jiyeon Lee, "South Korea Pulls Plug on Late-Night Adolescent Online Gamers," *CNN,* November 22, 2011.

17. "European Parliament Backs Initiative to Curb Digital Platform Addiction," *Digital Watch*, December 12, 2023; and "New EU Rules Needed to Address Digital Addiction," *European Parliament News*, December 12, 2023.

18. Clare Foran, "The Rise of the Internet-Addiction Industry," *The Atlantic*, November 5, 2015.

19. Kelvin Chan, "UK's New Online Safety Law Adds to Crackdown on Big Tech Companies," Associated Press, September 20, 2023; and David Shimer, "Germany Raids Homes of 36 People Accused of Hateful Postings over Social Media," *New York Times*, June 20, 2017.

Chapter 9

1. Jeffrey A. Singer, "A Former Governor Sees Things the Way Doctors Do," *InsideSources*, March 27, 2019.

2. Maia Szalavitz, *Undoing Drugs: The Untold Story of Harm Reduction and the Future of Addiction* (New York: Hachette Book Group, 2021); and Morgan Godvin, "On Drugs and Harm Reduction with Maia Szalavitz," *JSTOR Daily*, August 18, 2022.

3. Russell Newcombe, "High Time for Harm Reduction," *DrugLink*, January/February 1987.

4. Godvin, "On Drugs and Harm Reduction." Maia Szalavitz attributed the quote attributed to Margaret Thatcher in an interview.

5. "Drug Paraphernalia Fast Facts," Department of Justice, National Drug Intelligence Center; Jeffrey A. Singer and Sophia Heimowitz, "Drug Paraphernalia Laws Undermine Harm Reduction," Cato Institute Policy Analysis no. 929, June 7, 2022; and Jeffrey A. Singer, "Why Not Legalize All Drug Testing Equipment?," *Cato at Liberty* (blog), Cato Institute, August 1, 2023.

6. Katie Meyer, "Kenney: No More Arrests for Possession of Fentanyl Test Strips," *WHYY*, August 2, 2021.

7. As of January 2024, every state and the District of Columbia have allowed users to possess fentanyl test strips except Idaho, Indiana, Iowa, North Dakota, and Texas. Carl Smith, "Fentanyl Test Strips Are an Easy Way to Save Lives," *Governing*, January 24, 2024.

8. "21 U.S. Code § 856—Maintaining Drug-Involved Premises," Legal Information Institute, Cornell Law School; and Singer, "Why Not Legalize All Drug Testing Equipment?"

9. "21 U.S. Code § 856—Maintaining Drug-Involved Premises."

10. Jeffrey A. Singer, "Overdose Prevention Centers: A Successful Strategy for Preventing Death and Disease," Cato Institute Briefing Paper no. 149, February 28, 2023; and Jeffrey A. Singer, "The 'Crack House Statute' Is Hurting the Homeless When We Most Need Them Helped," *DC Examiner*, April 2, 2020.

11. Indhu Rammohan et al., "Overdose Mortality Incidence and Supervised Consumption Services in Toronto, Canada: An Ecological Study and Spatial Analysis," *Lancet Public Health* 9, no. 2 (February 2024): e79–87.

12. Jeffrey A. Singer and Sofia Hamilton, "Expand Access to Methadone Treatment," Cato Institute Policy Analysis no. 960, September 7, 2023.

13. Tony Romm, "House Approves $1.7 Trillion Omnibus Bill amid GOP Objections, Sending it to Biden," *Washington Post,* December 23, 2022; Jeffrey A. Singer, "Congress Made It Easier to Treat Addiction but Harder to Treat Pain," *Cato at Liberty* (blog), Cato Institute, December 23, 2022; and Jeffrey A. Singer, "DEA Pumps the Brakes on Congress' Move to Increase Access to Addiction Treatment," *Cato at Liberty* (blog), Cato Institute, March 15, 2023.

14. Dave Kriegel, "JUUL Review: 6 Years Later," Vaping360, July 21, 2021; Konstantinos Farsalinos et al., "Patterns of Flavored E-Cigarette Use Among Adults Vapers in the USA: An Online Cross-Sectional Survey of 69,233 Participants," *Harm Reduction Journal* 20 (October 2023); and Jeffrey A. Singer, "The FDA Is on a Quest to Snuff Out Tobacco Harm-Reduction," *Cato at Liberty* (blog), Cato Institute, June 22, 2022.

15. "Sen. Chuck Schumer Calling for Federal Action to Crack Down on a Product Called 'Zyn,'" CBS News, January 21, 2024; Jeffrey A. Singer, "What Is Causing Nicotinophobia?," *Cato at Liberty* (blog), Cato Institute, January 23, 2024; and Jeffrey A. Singer, "Why Attack Tobacco-Harm Reduction?," *National Review,* February 1, 2024.

Chapter 10

1. "Tobacco," NHS Inform, last updated November 1, 2024.

2. Luca Paoletti et al., "Current Status of Tobacco Policy and Control," *Journal of Thoracic Imaging* 27, no. 4 (July 2012): 213–19.

3. Mike Stobbe, "U.S. Adult Cigarette Smoking Hits New All-Time Low," *PBS NewsHour,* April 27, 2023.

4. Ernie Mundell, "US Teen Smoking Rates Have Plummeted, with Fewer than 1% Now Daily Smokers," *Medical Xpress,* January 10, 2024.

5. Jeffrey A. Singer, "Why Attack Tobacco Harm Reduction?," *National Review,* February 1, 2024.

6. Erin Keely O'Brien et al., "U.S. Adults' Addiction and Harm Beliefs about Nicotine and Low Nicotine Cigarettes," *Preventive Medicine* 96 (December 27, 2016): 94–100.

7. "Nicotine 'No More Harmful to Health than Caffeine,'" Royal Society for Public Health, August 13, 2015.

8. NHS Inform, "Tobacco," last updated August 15, 2024.

9. "Nicotine: from Plants to People," PMI Science, January 23, 2020.

10. Steven E. Meredith et al., "Caffeine Use Disorder: A Comprehensive Review and Research Agenda," *Journal of Caffeine Research* 3, no. 3 (September 2013): 114–30.

11. Angel Carvajal-Oliveros et al., "Nicotine Suppresses Parkinson's Disease Like Phenotypes Induced by Synphilin-1 Overexpression in *Drosophila Melanogaster* by Increasing Tyrosine Hydroxylase and Dopamine Levels," *Scientific Reports* 11 (2021).

12. Kelsey Herbers, "Study Explores Nicotine Patch to Treat Late-life Depression," Vanderbilt University Medical Center News, October 15, 2020; Brad Rodu,

"Nicotine, Smokeless Tobacco and Tourette's Syndrome," *R Street*, February 23, 2017; Tom Valeo, "Study Finds Nicotine Safe, Helps in Alzheimer's, Parkinson's," *Tampa Bay Times*, April 17, 2014; Ana Sandoiu, "Nicotine May Help Treat Schizophrenia, Study Finds," Medical News Today, January 15, 2017; Maryka Quik, Kathryn O'Leary, and Caroline M. Tanner, "Nicotine and Parkinson's Disease; Implications for Therapy," *Movement Disorders* 23, no. 12 (September 15, 2008): 1641–52; P. Newhouse et al., "Nicotine Treatment of Mild Cognitive Impairment: a 6-month Double-Blind Pilot Clinical Trial," *Neurology* 78, no. 2 (January 10, 2012): 91–101; and "Clinical Trial: Nicotine Patch Shows Benefits in Mild Cognitive Impairment," American Academy of Neurology press release, January 9, 2012.

13. Peter Hajek et al., "A Randomized Trial of E-Cigarettes versus Nicotine-Replacement Therapy," *New England Journal of Medicine* 380, no. 7 (January 2019): 629–37.

14. Jamie Hartmann-Boyce et al., "Electronic Cigarettes for Smoking Cessation," *Cochrane Database of Systematic Reviews*, November 17, 2022.

15. Matthew J. Carpenter et al., "Effect of Unguided E-cigarette Provision on Uptake, Use, And Smoking Cessation among Adults Who Smoke in the USA: A Naturalistic, Randomised, Controlled Clinical Trial," *The Lancet*, August 15, 2023.

16. Reto Auer et al., "Electronic Nicotine-Delivery Systems for Smoking Cessation," *New England Journal of Medicine* 390, no. 7 (February 15, 2024): 601–10.

17. House Amendment to the Senate Amendment to H.R. 1865, December 16, 2019; "Federal Tobacco 21: The Law of the Land," Tobacco 21.

18. Natasha A. Sokol and Justin M. Feldman, "High School Seniors Who Used E-Cigarettes May Have Otherwise Been Cigarette Smokers: Evidence from Monitoring the Future (United States, 2009–2018)," *Nicotine & Tobacco Research* 23 no. 11 (November 2021): 1958–61.

19. Alex Norcia, "Teens Who Vape Would Be Smoking if Vapes Weren't Invented, Study Suggests," *Filter*, May 18, 2021.

20. "Youth and Tobacco Use," US Centers for Disease Control and Prevention, October 17, 2024.

21. Matt Stout and Victoria McGrane, "State Lawmakers Pass Nation's Toughest Restrictions on Sale of Flavored Tobacco and Vaping Products," *Boston Globe*, November 21, 2019; and Jeffrey A. Singer, "Massachusetts Legislators' Rush to Judgment on Vaping Will Cause More Harm," *National Interest*, November 25, 2019.

22. "FDA Issues Marketing Denial Orders for Approximately 6,500 Flavored E-Cigarette Products," US Food and Drug Administration.

23. "The Vaping Panic Is Out of Hand," *New York Daily News*, September 19, 2019.

24. Farsalinos et al., "Patterns of Flavored E-cigarette Use among Adult Vapers in the USA"; and Dave Kriegel, "Juul Review: 6 Years Later," *Vaping360*, July 21, 2021.

25. Jeffrey A. Singer, "The FDA Is on A Quest to Snuff Out Tobacco Harm-Reduction," *Cato at Liberty* (blog), Cato Institute, June 22, 2022; and Jennifer Maloney, "Why the FDA Banned Juul E-Cigarettes," *Wall Street Journal*, October 21, 2022.

26. Matthew Perrone, "E-Cigarettes Like Elf Bar Face FDA Ban on Teen Vaping Concerns," Associated Press, December 30, 2023.

27. Guy Bentley, "Cigarette Sales Increase as Vaping Bans Push People Back to Smoking," *Reason*, August 24, 2020.

28. "Introduction to Heated Tobacco Products," California Department of Public Health.

29. "FDA Authorizes Three New Heated Tobacco Products," US Food and Drug Administration, January 26, 2023.

30. Jacob Grier, "It's Not a Cigarette. It's Not a Vape. And It's Big in Japan.," *Reason*, January 9, 2024.

31. Guy Bentley, "Setting the Record Straight on Heated Tobacco Products," *Reason*, September 1, 2021.

32. Jenny Gesley, "European Union: Prohibition on Flavored Heated Tobacco Products Enters into Force," Library of Congress, January 2, 2023.

33. "FDA Authorizes Three New Heated Tobacco Products."

34. "History of Snus," Swedish Match.

35. Frazer Norwell, "What Is Snus and Why Do So Many Norwegians Use It?," *The Local*, June 28, 2021; "Legality of Snus in Switzerland: Legal Situation Explained," SnusHus, December 21, 2021; Jen Christensen, "Smokeless Tobacco Company Can Advertise Snus as Less Risky Than Cigarettes, FDA Says," CNN, October 22, 2019; "Canada Snus/Nicotine Pouches Regulation," SnusLine, September 19, 2023; "Smoking, Vaping, HTP, NRT and Snus in Australia," Global State of Tobacco Harm Reduction; "Smoking, Vaping, HTP, NRT and Snus in New Zealand," Global State of Tobacco Harm Reduction; and "Smoking, Vaping, HTP, NRT and Snus in United Kingdom," Global State of Tobacco Harm Reduction.

36. Karl E. Lund, Janne Scheffels, and Ann McNeill, "The Association between Use of Snus and Quit Rates for Smoking: Results from Seven Norwegian Cross-Sectional Studies," *Addiction* 106, no. 1 (January 2011): 162–67.

37. Elizabeth Clarke et al., "Snus: A Compelling Harm Reduction Alternative to Cigarettes," *Harm Reduction Journal* 16, no. 62 (2019).

38. "Sen. Chuck Schumer Calling for Federal Action to Crack Down on a Product Called 'Zyn,'" *CBS News*, January 21, 2024; and Alexander Hall and Alexa Moutevelis, "Experts Say Schumer Attack on Zyn Is 'Moral Panic' about Smoke-free Nicotine Products That Can Save Lives," Fox News, January 26, 2024.

39. Hall and Moutevelis, "Experts Say Schumer Attack on Zyn is 'Moral Panic.'"

40. Jan Birdsey et al., "Tobacco Product Use among U.S. Middle and High School Students—National Youth Tobacco Survey, 2023," *Morbidity and Mortality Weekly Report* 72, no. 44 (2023): 1173–82.

41. Frances M. Leslie, "Unique, Long-term Effects of Nicotine on Adolescent Brain," *Pharmacology Biochemistry and Behavior* 197 (October 2020); and Emily M. Castro, Shahrdad Lotfipour, and Emily M. Castro, "Nicotine on the Developing Brain," *Pharmacological Research* 190 (2023).

42. Yeyetzi C. Torres-Ugalde et al., "Caffeine Consumption in Children: Innocuous or Deleterious? A Systematic Review," *International Journal of Environmental*

Research and Public Health 17, no. 7 (2020): 2489; Claire McCarthy, "Alcohol Harms the Brain in Teen Years—Before and After That, Too," *Harvard Health Blog*, January 15, 2021; and "Caffeine and Kids," Columbia University Irving Medical Center, August 3, 2022.

43. "What Is Zyn and What Are Oral Nicotine Pouches?," Truth Initiative, June 7, 2024; and "Our Mission," Truth Initiative.

44. Policy analyst Michelle Minton claims that "Though concerns over e-cigarettes' long-term effects are reasonable, that is not the impetus behind the anti-e-cigarette movement. Rather . . . it is the consequence of those groups and individuals vested with the power and funding of the government seemingly prioritizing their organizational interests over public health." Michelle Minton, "Fear Profiteers: How E-cigarette Panic Benefits Health Activists," Competitive Enterprise Institute, December 2018, p. 7.

45. "Is Vaping Harmful?," Cancer Research UK, March 27, 2023; and Jeffrey A. Singer, "What Is Causing Nicotinophobia?," *Cato at Liberty* (blog), Cato Institute, January 23, 2024.

Chapter 11

1. Yu-Jen Shih, Wei-Ning Chang, and Shan-Wei Yang, "Heroin-Induced Osteoporosis Presented with Bilateral Femoral Neck Insufficiency Fractures in a Male Adult: a Case Report," *BMC Musculoskeletal Disorders* 24, no. 296 (2023).

2. "Cocaine/Fentanyl Combination in Pennsylvania," Drug Enforcement Administration, February 2018; Scott Maucione, "Fentanyl Mixed with Cocaine or Meth Is Driving the 4th Wave of the Overdose Crisis," *NPR*, September 14, 2023; and "San Fernando Valley Man Who Sold Counterfeit Prescription Pills Containing Fentanyl Admits Causing Overdose Death of U.S. Marine," US Department of Justice, April 15, 2022.

3. "5 Things to Know About Naloxone: Naloxone Is One Important Step," US Centers for Disease Control and Prevention, May 2, 2024; and "Naloxone DrugFacts," National Institute on Drug Abuse, January 11, 2022.

4. "Guidelines for the Psychosocially Assisted Pharmacological Treatment of Opioid Dependence," World Health Organization.

5. "Infographic. Availability of Naloxone Take-Home Naloxone Programmes in Europe," European Union Drugs Agency, December 14, 2021.

6. "U.S. Surgeon General's Advisory on Naloxone and Opioid Overdose," US Department of Health and Human Services, April 8, 2022; Jeffrey A. Singer, "To Save Lives, Make Naloxone an Over-the-Counter Drug," *Reason*, April 27, 2018; and Jeffrey A. Singer, "The FDA Bends Over Backwards to Get Drug Makers to Ask Them to Make Naloxone OTC," *Cato at Liberty* (blog), Cato Institute, January 18, 2019.

7. Penny Timms, "Naloxone: Heroin Overdose Cure to Be Available Over the Counter as Drug Makes a Comeback," *ABC News*, December 15, 2015; Susanna Ronconi, "Learning from Italy's Lead on Naloxone," Open Society

Foundations, March 30, 2017; and "Infographic. Availability of Take-Home Naloxone Programmes in Europe," European Union Drugs Agency, December 14, 2021.

8. Julie Wernau, "FDA Makes Overdose-Reversal Drug Narcan Available Over-the-Counter," *Wall Street Journal*, March 29, 2023; and Jeffrey A. Singer, "FDA to Finally Let People Get Naloxone Without a Prescription," *Cato at Liberty* (blog), Cato Institute, March 29, 2023.

9. "History: 1975–1980," Drug Enforcement Administration, pp. 44–45.

10. Jeffrey A. Singer and Sophia Heimowitz, "Drug Paraphernalia Laws Undermine Harm Reduction," Cato Institute Policy Analysis no. 929, June 7, 2022.

11. Kyle Jaeger, "Minnesota Lawmakers Vote to Legalize Drug Paraphernalia, Residue, Testing and Syringe Services," Marijuana Moment, May 17, 2023; and Jeffrey A. Singer, "Minnesota Repeals Its Drug Paraphernalia Laws," *Cato at Liberty* (blog), Cato Institute, May 24, 2023.

12. Gregg S. Gonsalves and Forrest W. Crawford, "Dynamics of the HIV Outbreak and Response in Scott County, Indiana, 2011–2015: A Modeling Study," *Lancet HIV* 5, no. 10 (October 2018): e569–e577.

13. Tyler S. Bartholomew et al., "Reduction in Injection Risk Behaviors after Implementation of a Syringe Services Program, in Miami, Florida," *Journal of Substance Abuse Treatment* 127 (August 2021): 108344.

14. "Fact Sheet: Syringe Services Programs in California: An Overview," California Department of Public Health, Center for Infectious Diseases, Office of AIDS, September 2022.

15. K. J. Bornstein et al., "Hospital Admissions among People Who Inject Opioids Following Syringe Services Program Implementation," *Harm Reduction Journal* 17, no. 30 (May 12, 2020).

16. "Drug Paraphernalia Fast Facts," National Drug Intelligence Center, Department of Justice.

17. Nicholas Lassi, "Strengthening Pill Press Control to Combat Fentanyl: Legislative and Law Enforcement Imperatives," *Exploratory Research in Clinical and Social Pharmacy* 11 (September 2023): Discussion, 4.1; and "21 U.S. Code § 830—Regulation of Listed Chemicals and Certain Machines," Legal Information Institute, Cornell Law School.

18. Ariz. Rev. Stat. § 13–3415, sections A and B. "Possession, Manufacture, Delivery and Advertisement of Drug Paraphernalia; Classification; Civil Forfeiture; Factors; Definitions."

19. Drug Paraphernalia Control Act, 720 Ill. Comp. Stat. 600/2. Section 2(d)(3).

20. Rick Noack, "Music Festivals Are Offering to Test the Safety of People's Drugs, and Police Increasingly Like the Idea," *Washington Post*, January 4, 2019.

21. J. J. Palamar et al., "Drug Checking at Dance Festivals: A Review with Recommendations to Increase Generalizability of Findings," *Experimental and Clinical Psychopharmacology* 29, no. 3 (2021): 229–35; Jamie Doward, "Testing Drugs at Festivals Is 'a Lifesaver,' Study Finds," *The Guardian* (London), December 8, 2018; and "DanceSafe."

22. Fiona Catherine Measham, "Drug Safety Testing, Disposals and Dealing in an English Field: Exploring the Operational and Behavioural Outcomes of

the UK's First Onsite 'Drug Checking' Service," *International Journal of Drug Policy* 67 (May 2019): 102–07.

23. "Legality of Drug Checking Equipment in the United States: August 2022 Update," Network for Public Health Law.

24. Jeffrey A. Singer, "Fentanyl Test Strips Save Lives, Yet Most States Ban Them as 'Drug Paraphernalia,'" *Cato at Liberty* (blog), Cato Institute, January 19, 2023.

25. Margaret Osborne, "Lifesaving Fentanyl Test Strips Are Being Legalized in More States," *Smithsonian*, June 9, 2023.

26. "DEA Reports Widespread Threat of Fentanyl Mixed with Xylazine," Drug Enforcement Administration, Public Safety Alert.

27. "Characterization of Xylazine Test Strips for Use in Drug Checking," Center for Forensic Science Research and Education, January 18, 2023.

28. Jeffrey A. Singer, "Why Not Legalize All Drug Testing Equipment?," *Cato at Liberty* (blog), Cato Institute, August 1, 2023.

29. Singer and Heimowitz, "Drug Paraphernalia Laws Undermine Harm Reduction."

30. "Expanding Naloxone Use Could Reduce Drug Overdose Deaths and Save Lives," Centers for Disease Control and Prevention, press release, April 24, 2015; and Jeffrey A. Singer, "Harm Reduction: Shifting from a War on Drugs to a War on Drug-Related Deaths," Cato Institute Policy Analysis no. 858, December 13, 2018.

31. "Syringe Services Programs," Centers for Disease Control and Prevention, February 8, 2024.

32. See, for example, David P. Wilson et al., "The Cost-Effectiveness of Harm Reduction," *International Journal on Drug Policy* 26, no. S1 (February 2015): S5–11 ("not only did [syringe service programs (SSPs)] reduce the incidence of HIV by up to 74 percent over a 10-year period in Australia but they were cost-saving [to the government] and had a return on investment of between $1.3 and $5.5 for every $1 spent"); Hrishikesh K. Belani and Peter A. Muennig, "Cost-Effectiveness of Needle and Syringe Exchange for the Prevention of HIV in New York City," *Journal of HIV/AIDS & Social Services* 7, no. 3 (September 15, 2008): 229–40 (SSPs "reduced HIV treatment costs by $325,000 per HIV case averted, and averted 4–7 HIV infections per 1000 clients, producing a net cost savings"); Trang Q. Nguyen et al., "Syringe Exchange in the United States: A National Level Economic Evaluation of Hypothetical Increases in Investment," *AIDS and Behavior* 18, no. 11 (November 2014): 2144–55 ("With an annual $10 to $50 million [SSP] funding increase, 194–816 HIV infections would be averted (cost per infection averted $51,601–$61,302)"); Bureau for Public Health, "White Paper: The Need for Harm Reduction Programs in West Virginia," West Virginia Department of Health and Human Resources, November 6, 2017 (citing studies estimating that SSPs could avert 15 to 33 percent of HIV cases, with a cost savings of between $20,947 and $34,278 per HIV case averted); Stephen C. Ijioma et al., "Cost-Effectiveness of Syringe Service Programs, Medications for Opioid Use Disorder, and Combination Programs in Hepatitis C Harm Reduction among Opioid Injection Drug Users: A Public Payer Perspective

Using a Decision Tree," *Journal of Managed Care & Specialty Pharmacy* 27, no. 2 (February 1, 2021): 137–46 (incremental cost savings of $363,821 per hepatitis C case averted by SSPs alone); and "Syringe Services Programs."

33. Bornstein et al., "Hospital Admissions among People Who Inject Opioids," p. 30; and "Syringe Services Programs—A Critical Public Health Intervention," Office of the Assistant Secretary for Health, July 30, 2019.

34. Kate Dolan et al., "Drug Consumption Facilities in Europe and the Establishment of Supervised Injecting Centres in Australia," *Drug and Alcohol Review* 19, no. 3 (2000): 337–46.

35. Alex H. Kral et al., "Transition from Injecting Opioids to Smoking Fentanyl in San Francisco, California," *Drug and Alcohol Dependence* 227 (October 1, 2021); Daniel Ciccarone, "Heroin Smoking Is Not Common in the United States," *JAMA Neurology* 74, no. 4 (March 11, 2019): 508; and Erika Edwards, "Once Feared, Illicit Fentanyl Is Now a Drug of Choice for Many Opioid Users," *NBC News*, August 7, 2022. Heroin smoking has historically been more popular in Europe. In the United States, heroin and fentanyl users are increasingly switching from injecting to smoking or other forms of inhalation. Some switch because they are running out of injectable veins. Others view inhalation as a form of harm reduction because it avoids using or sharing contaminated needles that risk transmission of HIV, hepatitis, and other infections. Some believe they can more carefully calibrate the dose of fentanyl by inhaling until they achieve the desired effect and thus reduce the risk of overdosing. Finally, because illicit fentanyl often is in pill form, users sometimes find it easier to crush and smoke the fentanyl than to liquefy and inject it.

36. Jeffrey A. Singer, "Harm Reduction: Shifting from a War on Drugs to a War on Drug-Related Deaths," Cato Institute Policy Analysis no. 858, December 13, 2018; and "Supervised Consumption and Overdose Prevention Sites," Vancouver Coastal Health.

37. "What Is the Effectiveness of Supervised Injection Services?," Ontario HIV Treatment Network *Rapid Review* no. 83, May 2014; Steven Petrar et al., "Injection Drug Users' Perceptions Regarding Use of a Medically Supervised Safer Injecting Facility," *Addictive Behaviors* 32, no. 5 (May 2007): 1088–93; and Kora DeBeck et al., "Injection Drug Use Cessation and Use of North America's First Medically Supervised Safer Injecting Facility," *Drug and Alcohol Dependence* 113, nos. 2–3 (January 15, 2011): 172–76.

38. Dagmar Hedrich et al., "Drug Consumption Rooms," joint report by the European Harm Reduction Network and the European Monitoring Centre for Drugs and Drug Addiction, December 2023; Jeffrey A. Singer, "Overdose Prevention Centers: A Successful Strategy for Preventing Death and Disease," Cato Institute briefing paper no. 149, February 28, 2023; and Anna Betts, "Providence Officials Approve Overdose Prevention Center," *New York Times*, February 4, 2024.

39. Jeffrey A. Singer, "Tragedy Strikes at Canadian Overdose Prevention Center Despite Staff Efforts," *Cato at Liberty* (blog), Cato Institute, October 8, 2024; and "Client Dies After Visiting London's Carepoint Facility," CTV News London, October 3, 2024.

40. "21 U.S. Code § 856 - Maintaining Drug-Involved Premises," Legal Information Institute, Cornell Law School.

41. Emerson Soto, "OnPoint NYC, Operators of the Nation's First Supervised Consumption Centers, Announces That It Has Intervened in Over 1,000 Overdoses," OnPoint NYC, August 9, 2023; and Jeffrey A. Singer, "New York City's Two Overdose Prevention Centers Saved One Thousand Lives Since They Opened. Will The Feds Reward Them by Shutting Them Down?," *Cato at Liberty* (blog), Cato Institute, August 9, 2023.

42. Katie Mulvaney, "RI Gov. McKee Signs Legislation Allowing Safe-Injection Sites into Law," *Providence Journal*, July 7, 2021; and Jeffrey A. Singer, "Rhode Island Makes Harm Reduction History by Legalizing Safe Consumption Sites," *Cato at Liberty* (blog), Cato Institute, July 8, 2021.

43. Alexander Castro, "First State-Regulated Overdose Prevention Center Could Open by Summer in Providence," *Rhode Island Current*, February 2, 2024.

44. Lesley McClurg, "California Debates Opening Supervised Sites for People to Use Drugs," *NPR*, May 23, 2022.

45. Nora D. Volkow and A. Thomas McLellan, "Opioid Abuse in Chronic Pain— Misconceptions and Mitigation Strategies," *New England Journal of Medicine* 374 (March 31, 2016): 1253–63; Gavan P. McNally et al., "Pathways to the Persistence of Drug Use Despite Its Adverse Consequences," *Molecular Psychiatry* 28 (2023): 2228–37; and Jeffrey A. Singer, "The March Toward a Pre-Modern Approach to the Treatment of Pain Continues, Undeterred by Science," *Cato at Liberty* (blog), Cato Institute, August 12, 2019.

46. *Merriam-Webster*, s.v. "agonist." See also John Strang et al., "Opioid Use Disorder," *Nature Reviews Disease Primers* 6, no. 3 (2020).

47. Ilene B. Anderson and Thomas E. Kearney, "Use of Methadone," *Western Journal of Medicine* 172, no. 1 (January 2000): 43–46.

48. R. P. Mattick et al., "Buprenorphine Maintenance versus Placebo or Methadone Maintenance for Opioid Dependence," Cochrane, February 6, 2014.

49. Adam N. Peddicord, Chris Bush, and Crystal Cruze, "A Comparison of Suboxone and Methadone in the Treatment of Opiate Addiction," *Journal of Addiction Research and Therapy* 6, no. 248 (November 27, 2015).

50. Richard P. Mattick et al., "Buprenorphine Maintenance versus Placebo or Methadone Maintenance for Opioid Dependence," *Cochrane Database of Systematic Reviews* 2 (February 6, 2014): 248; and Louisa Degenhardt et al., "Buprenorphine versus Methadone for the Treatment of Opioid Dependence: A Systematic Review and Meta-Analysis of Randomised and Observational Studies," *Lancet Psychiatry* 10, no. 6 (June 2023): 386–402.

51. Silvia Minozzi et al., "Oral Naltrexone Maintenance Treatment for Opioid Dependence," *Cochrane Database of Systematic Reviews* 4 (April 13, 2011): CD001333.

52. Sarah E. Wakeman et al., "Comparative Effectiveness of Different Treatment Pathways for Opioid Use Disorder," *JAMA Network Open* 3, no. 2 (February 5, 2020).

53. Marica Ferri, Marina Davoli, and Carlo A. Perucci, "Heroin Maintenance for Chronic Heroin-Dependent Individuals," *Cochrane Database of Systematic Reviews* (December 7, 2011): CD003410.

54. Drug Addiction Treatment Act of 2000, H. R. 2634, 106th Cong., 2nd Sess. (2000); Jeffrey A. Singer, "Will Congress Finally X-Out the 'X' Waiver," *Cato at Liberty* (blog), Cato Institute, July 16, 2019; and Joyce Frieden, "HHS Loosens Rules for Prescribing Buprenorphine," *Medpage Today*, April 27, 2021.

55. Noah Weiland, "More Doctors Can Now Prescribe a Key Opioid Treatment. Will It Help?," *New York Times*, March 3, 2023; "Buprenorphine," Substance Abuse and Mental Health Services Administration, U.S. Department of Health and Human Services, updated March 28, 2024; Jeffrey A. Singer, "Congress Made It Easier to Treat Addiction but Harder to Treat Pain," *Cato at Liberty* (blog), Cato Institute, December 23, 2022; and Jeffrey A. Singer, "DEA Pumps the Brakes on Congress' Move to Increase Access to Addiction Treatment," *Cato at Liberty* (blog), Cato Institute, March 15, 2023.

56. Lev Facher, "Providers Still Hesitate to Prescribe Buprenorphine for Addiction, Despite 'X-Waiver' Removal," *STAT News*, July 21, 2023.

57. A. J. Reid Finlayson, Jeffrey A. Singer, and Peter R. Martin, "The DEA's War on Addiction Doctors," *KevinMD*, December 19, 2023.

58. Richard A. Rettig and Adam Yarmolinsky, eds., *Federal Regulation of Methadone Treatment* (Washington: National Academy Press, 1995), Google Books edition, chap. 5, pp. 120–44.

59. Comprehensive Drug Abuse Prevention and Control Act of 1970, Pub. L. No. 91-513, 84 Stat. 1241 (1970), Title I, Section 4, "Medical Treatment of Narcotic Addition," quoted in Rettig and Yarmolinsky, eds., *Federal Regulation of Methadone Treatment*, Executive Summary, p. 2.

60. Sheri Doyle, "Federal Agencies Have Substantial Authority to Boost Methadone Access," Pew Charitable Trusts, August 11, 2022.

61. Jeffrey H. Samet et al., "Methadone in Primary Care–One Small Step for Congress, One Giant Leap for Addiction Treatment," *New England Journal of Medicine* 379, no. 1 (2018): 7–8.

62. Jeffrey A. Singer and Sofia Hamilton, "Expand Access to Methadone Treatment," Cato Institute Policy Analysis no. 960, September 7, 2023.

63. Jeffrey A. Singer, "The Modernizing Opioid Treatment Access Act Is a Good Step in the Right Direction, But It Should Go Further," *Cato at Liberty* (blog), Cato Institute, March 20, 2023; and Jeffrey A. Singer, "First Serious Effort in Years to Expand Access to Methadone Treatment," *Cato at Liberty* (blog), Cato Institute, December 7, 2023.

64. Chris Roberts, "Drug Users Are Being Sentenced to Forced Rehab. But Does It Work?," *Vice*, September 17, 2021.

65. Jeffrey A. Singer," Oregon Lawmakers Roll Back New Drug War Strategy and Revert to Decades-Old Approach Linked to Soaring Overdose Deaths," *Cato at Liberty* (blog), Cato Institute, March 2, 2024; and "Staff Measure Summary," 82nd Oregon Legislative Assembly, 2024 Regular Session, February 27, 2024.

66. "Involuntary Commitment for Substance Abuse," The Action Lab at the Center for Health and Policy Law, Data Dashboard, Northeastern University.

67. John Tierney, "The Rational Choices of Crack Addicts," *New York Times*, September 16, 2013; and German Lopez, "Watch: A Neuroscientist Debunks Common Beliefs about Drug Addiction," *Vox*, September 18, 2014.

68. Jake Flanagin, "The Surprising Failures of 12 Steps," *The Atlantic*, March 25, 2014; William Wagner, "Psychologist Stanton Peele on Treatment Beyond 12 Steps," *Treatment Magazine*, July 10, 2020; and Maia Szalavitz, "Does Addiction Treatment Require a Higher Power?," *NPR*, May 1, 2016; and Maia Szalavitz, "After 75 Years of Alcoholics Anonymous, It's Time to Admit We Have a Problem," *Pacific Standard*, updated June 14, 2017.

69. Sarah E. Wakeman, "Why Involuntary Treatment for Addiction Is a Dangerous Idea," *STAT News*, April 25, 2023.

70. Claudia Rafful et al., "Increased Non-Fatal Overdose Risk Associated with Involuntary Drug Treatment in a Longitudinal Study with People Who Inject Drugs," *Addiction* 113, no. 6 (2018): 1056–63.

71. D. Werb et al., "The Effectiveness of Compulsory Drug Treatment: A Systematic Review," *International Journal of Drug Policy* 28 (February 2016): 1–9.

72. "An Assessment of Opioid-Related Deaths in Massachusetts (2013–2014)," Commonwealth of Massachusetts, Executive Office of Health and Human Services, Department of Public Health, September 2016.

73. Martin P. Wegman et al., "Relapse to Opioid Use in Opioid-Dependent Individuals Released from Compulsory Drug Detention Centres Compared with Those from Voluntary Methadone Treatment Centres in Malaysia: a T-Arm, Prospective Observational Study," *Lancet Global Health* 5, no. 2 (February 2017): e198–e207.

74. Karen Giang et al., "Risk Mitigation Guidance and Safer Supply Prescribing among Young People Who Use Drugs in the Context of COVID-19 and Overdose Emergencies," *International Journal on Drug Policy* 115 (2023): 104023.

75. Jan Hoffman, "Fentanyl Tainted Pills Bought on Social Media Cause Youth Drug Deaths to Soar," *New York Times*, May 19, 2022.

76. "Safe Supply Work Group: Preliminary Report," Washington State Legislature, December 1, 2023; Benedikt Fischer and Tessa Robinson, "'Safer Drug Supply Measures in Canada to Reduce the Drug Overdose Fatality Toll: Clarifying Concepts, Practices and Evidence Within a Public Health Intervention Framework,'" *Journal of Studies on Alcohol and Drugs* 84, no. 6 (2023): 801–07; Giang et al., "Risk Mitigation Guidance"; Marilou Gagnon et al., "Impact of Safer Supply Programs on Injection Practices: Client and Provider Experiences in Ontario, Canada," *Harm Reduction Journal* 20, no. 81 (June 28, 2023); and Hai V. Nguyen et al., "British Columbia's Safer Opioid Supply Policy and Opioid Outcomes," *JAMA Internal Medicine* 184, no. 3 (2024): 256–64.

Chapter 12

1. Steven J. Scheinman, Patrick Fleming, and Kellyann Niotis, "Oath Taking at U.S. and Canadian Medical School Ceremonies: Historical Perspectives, Current Practices, and Future Considerations," *Academic Medicine* 93, no. 9 (September 2018): 1301–06; and "Physician Oaths," Association of American Physicians and Surgeons.

2. Declaration of Geneva: The "Modern Hippocratic Oath," World Medical Association.

204 YOUR BODY, YOUR HEALTH CARE

3. "The Hippocratic Oath: Modern Version," NOVA PBS.
4. "What Do Medical Students Hope to Remember about their White Coat Ceremonies?," Gold Foundation, September 12, 2013.
5. Scheinman et al., "Oath Taking at U.S. and Canadian Medical School Ceremonies: Historical Perspectives, Current Practices, and Future Considerations," *Academic Medicine* 93, no. 9 (September 2018): 1301–06.
6. Nonny Onyekweli, "A Medical School Class Thought the Hippocratic Oath Fell Flat. So They Wrote Their Own Script," *Inspired Life* (blog), *Washington Post*, September 26, 2020.
7. "Modern Hippocratic Oath Holds the Underlying Values of Medicine in a Digital World," David Geffen School of Medicine, UCLA, July 13, 2018; and Stacy Weiner, "The Solemn Truth about Medical Oaths," *AAMC*, July 10, 2018.
8. "Physician Oaths," Association of American Physicians and Surgeons.
9. "A Modern Hippocratic Oath by Dr. Louis Lasagna," Association of American Physicians and Surgeons.
10. Jeffrey A. Singer, "A Hippocratic Oath for a Free Society," Cato Institute (visual feature), May 8, 2023.

INDEX

Note: Information in figures is indicated by *f*; n designates a numbered note.

ABOUT THE AUTHOR

Jeffrey A. Singer is a senior fellow at the Cato Institute and works in the Department of Health Policy Studies. He is president emeritus and founder of Valley Surgical Clinics Ltd., the largest and oldest group private surgical practice in Arizona, and has been in private practice as a general surgeon for more than 35 years.

He is also a visiting fellow at the Goldwater Institute in Phoenix. Singer is a member of the Board of Scientific Advisors of the American Council on Science and Health. From 1994 to 2016, he was a regular contributor to *Arizona Medicine*, the journal of the Arizona Medical Association. He served on the advisory board for the Council of the Center for Political Thought and Leadership at Arizona State University from 2014 to 2018. He writes and speaks extensively on regional and national public policy, with a specific focus on the areas of health care policy and the harmful effects of drug prohibition.

He received his BA from Brooklyn College (City University of New York) and his MD from New York Medical College. He is a fellow of the American College of Surgeons.

ABOUT THE CATO INSTITUTE

Founded in 1977, the Cato Institute is a public policy research foundation dedicated to broadening the parameters of policy debate to allow consideration of more options that are consistent with the principles of limited government, individual liberty, and peace. The Institute is named for *Cato's Letters*, libertarian pamphlets that were widely read in the American colonies in the early 18th century and played a major role in laying the philosophical foundation for the American Revolution.

The Cato Institute undertakes an extensive publications program on the complete spectrum of policy issues. Books, monographs, and shorter studies are commissioned to examine the federal budget, Social Security, regulation, military spending, international trade, and myriad other issues. Major policy conferences are held throughout the year.

In order to maintain its independence, the Cato Institute accepts no government funding. Contributions are received from foundations, corporations, and individuals, and other revenue is generated from the sale of publications. The Institute is a nonprofit, tax-exempt, educational foundation under Section 501(c)3 of the Internal Revenue Code.

CATO INSTITUTE
1000 Massachusetts Ave. NW
Washington, DC 20001
www.cato.org